COMPREHENSIVE BONE HEALTH STRATEGIES

SCIENCE BASED HOLISTIC APPROACH

DR. K.D. CHRISTENSEN

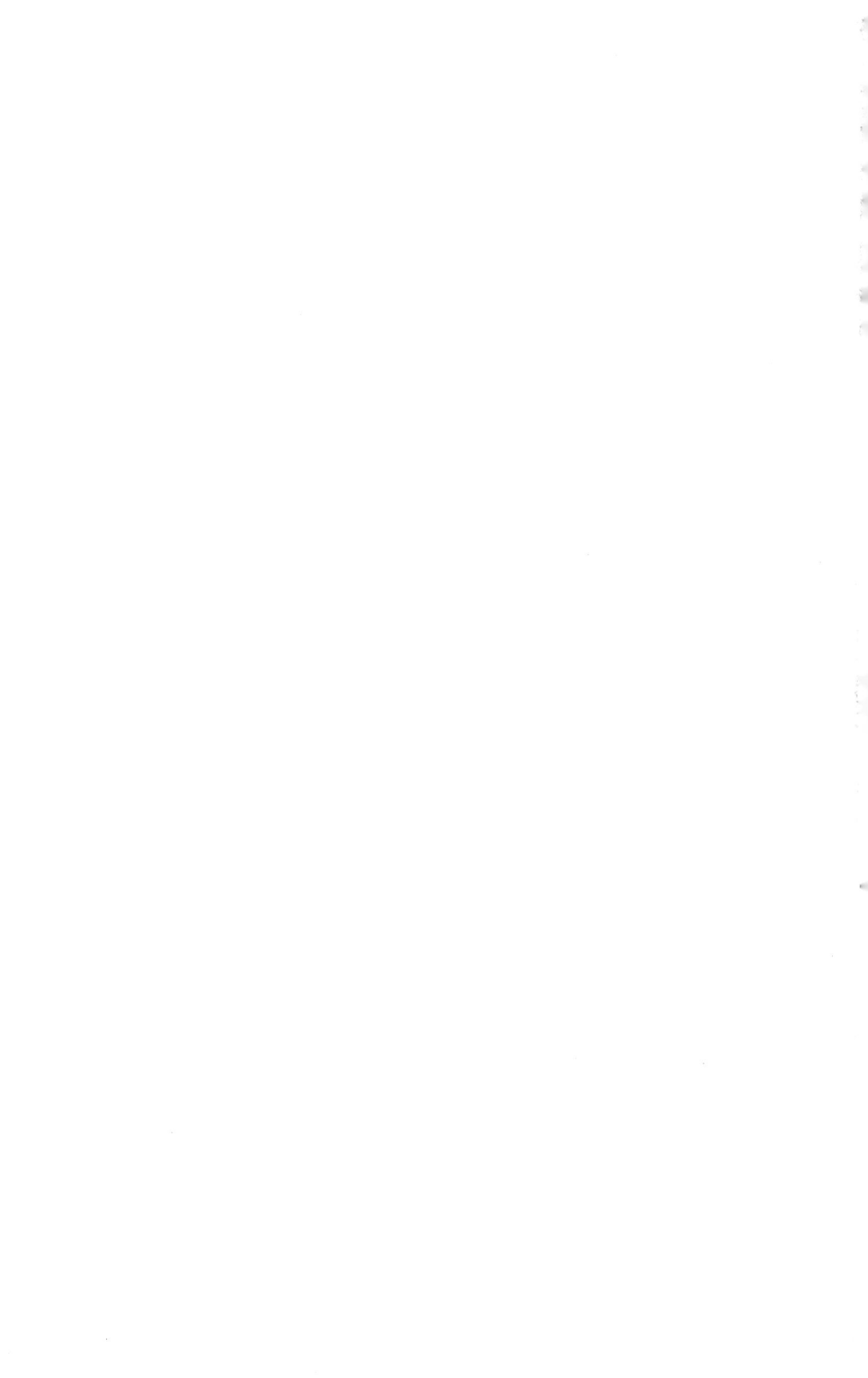

CONTENTS

Introduction — 7

1. UNDERSTANDING BONE HEALTH — 11
   1.1 Anatomy of Bones: What You Need to Know — 11
   1.2 Osteoporosis and Osteopenia: Differences and Diagnoses — 14
   1.3 Arthritis: Types, Symptoms, and Bone Health Impact — 17
   1.4 The Science Behind Bone Density — 20

2. MEDICAL OPTIONS AND EXPLANATIONS — 25
   2.1 Bone Density Scans: What They Reveal — 25
   2.2 Prescription Medications: Benefits and Side Effects — 28
   2.3 Interpreting Your Bone Health Report — 30
   2.4 Discussing Treatment Plans with Your Doctor — 33
   2.5 Non-Pharmaceutical Interventions for Bone Health — 36

3. NUTRITIONAL GUIDANCE FOR BONE HEALTH — 39
   3.1 Understanding Calcium and Its Role in Bone Health — 39
   3.2 Vitamin D: The Sunshine Vitamin's Role in Bone Density — 42
   3.3 Protein and Bone Health: How Much Do You Need? — 44
   3.4 Foods to Boost Bone Health: A Comprehensive List — 47
   3.5 Meal Plans for Optimal Bone Health — 49

4. SUPPLEMENT INFORMATION — 53
   4.1 Essential Supplements for Bone Health: What to Take — 53
   4.2 Calcium Supplements: Dosages and Best Practices — 57

4.3 Vitamin D Supplements: Choosing the Right One	60
4.4 Understanding Multivitamins and Their Impact on Bone Health	63

5. DETAILED EXERCISE ROUTINES — 67
   5.1 Bone-Building Workouts: Introduction and Benefits — 67
   5.2 Beginner Exercise Routines: Step-by-Step Guide — 70
   5.3 Intermediate Exercise Routines: Step-by-Step Guide — 76
   5.4 Advanced Exercise Routines: Step-by-Step Guide — 84

6. PRACTICAL TIPS AND STRATEGIES FOR DAILY MANAGEMENT — 91
   6.1 Setting Realistic Goals for Bone Health — 91
   6.2 Daily Habits for Stronger Bones — 94
   6.3 Tracking Your Progress: Tools and Techniques — 96
   6.4 Staying Motivated: Tips for Consistency — 99
   6.5 Fall Prevention: Safe Practices for Home and Outdoors — 101

7. HOLISTIC HEALTH APPROACH — 105
   7.1 Integrating Diet and Exercise for Bone Health — 105
   7.2 Stress Management Techniques for Better Bone Health — 107
   7.3 Smoking Cessation and Bone Health — 109
   7.4 The Role of Sleep in Bone Health — 110
   7.5 Reducing Alcohol Intake for Stronger Bones — 113

8. PERSONAL STORIES AND TESTIMONIALS — 117
   8.1 Overcoming Osteoporosis: Jane's Story — 117
   8.2 From Diagnosis to Recovery: Mark's Journey — 119
   8.3 Staying Active with Arthritis: Linda's Experience — 121
   8.4 The Power of Nutrition: Rachel's Transformation — 123
   8.5 Holistic Health Success: John's Testimony — 125

9. ADDRESSING COMMON PAIN POINTS AND QUESTIONS — 129
   9.1 Safe Exercises to Prevent Falls — 129
   9.2 Navigating Nutritional Needs Without Confusion — 131
   9.3 Managing Limited Mobility in Exercise Routines — 133

	9.4 Effective Supplementation: What Actually Works	136
	9.5 Staying Consistent: Overcoming Motivation Barriers	138
10.	INTERACTIVE ELEMENTS AND TOOLS	141
	10.1 Exercise Tracking Charts	141
	10.2 Meal Planning Templates	144
	10.3 Supplement Dosage Schedules	150
	10.4 Weekly Progress Journals	153
	Conclusion	159
	References	163

INTRODUCTION

Years ago, a dear patient named Margaret shared with me her struggles. She had always been active, enjoying long walks and gardening. But as she entered her seventies, she began to experience severe joint pain and frequent falls. Her once-vibrant lifestyle diminished. She was diagnosed with osteoporosis and arthritis. Margaret's story is not unique, but it serves as a powerful reminder of the importance of bone health, especially for seniors.

As we age, maintaining strong and healthy bones becomes increasingly vital. Bone health impacts our mobility, independence, and overall quality of life. For seniors, the risk of osteoporosis and arthritis can lead to severe consequences, including fractures and chronic pain. These conditions can limit daily activities and reduce the ability to enjoy life fully. Addressing bone health proactively is crucial for preventing these issues and ensuring a better quality of life in later years.

The purpose of this book is to provide you with a science-based, holistic approach to bone health. Here, we will explore not only the medical options available but also the lifestyle changes, nutritional guidance, and exercise routines that can make a significant difference. My vision is to offer you practical tips and strategies that are easy to understand and implement. By following the guidance in this book, you can take control of your bone health and improve your overall well-being.

What sets this book apart is its comprehensive approach. We will delve into personal stories and testimonials to illustrate the real-life impact of bone health issues and their solutions. You will find detailed exercise routines specifically designed for seniors, nutritional advice to support bone strength, and information on supplements that can aid in maintaining healthy bones. Moreover, we will explore medical options and provide explanations to help you make informed decisions. This holistic approach ensures that all aspects of bone health are covered, giving you a complete guide to improving and maintaining your bone health.

The book is structured to provide you with a clear and organized path to better bone health. We will begin with an understanding of bone health and its importance for seniors. Next, we will explore medical options and their benefits. Following this, we will dive into lifestyle changes and how they can positively impact your bone health. Detailed exercise routines will be provided, along with nutritional guidance and supplement information. Practical tips and strategies will be interwoven throughout the chapters, giving you actionable steps to take. Each chapter builds on the previous one, ensuring a cohesive and comprehensive guide.

Allow me to introduce myself. I am Dr. K.D. Christensen, a retired Sports Chiropractor certified in Rehabilitation with over 40 years of experience. Throughout my career, I have worked with countless patients to improve their bone health and overall well-being. My extensive experience and dedication to helping seniors maintain their mobility and independence have led me to write this book. I aim to share the knowledge and insights I have gained over the years to help you achieve better bone health.

As you read this book, expect to find clear, actionable advice backed by scientific research. You will gain a more in-depth understanding of bone health and learn practical steps to improve it. Whether you are dealing with osteoporosis, arthritis, or simply want to maintain strong bones as you age, this book will provide you with the tools you need. Engage with the content, try the exercises, and incorporate the nutritional and lifestyle recommendations into your daily routine. Your commitment to improving your bone health will lead to a more active and fulfilling life.

I encourage you to approach this book with an open mind and a willingness to make positive changes. The journey to better bone health is a continuous one, but with the right knowledge and tools, it is entirely achievable. Take the first step today, and commit to prioritizing your bone health. Together, we will navigate the path to stronger, healthier bones, and a better quality of life in your senior years.

1

UNDERSTANDING BONE HEALTH

When I first met Jack, he was a robust 72-year-old who had always prided himself on his physical fitness. Yet, a minor fall left him with a fractured hip, a stark reminder of how fragile our bones can become with age. This incident underscored the critical need to understand bone health, particularly for seniors. As we delve into this chapter, we'll explore the anatomy of bones, their functions, and the processes that keep them healthy. Understanding these foundational aspects is the first step towards ensuring robust bone health as we age.

1.1 ANATOMY OF BONES: WHAT YOU NEED TO KNOW

Bones are marvels of nature, intricate in their design and vital in their function. They are not just rigid structures, but dynamic organs that play several crucial roles in our bodies. To appreciate the importance of bone health, one must first understand the basic structure and composition of bones. Bones are composed of several different layers and types of tissue, each serving a unique purpose.

The outermost layer is known as the periosteum. This dense, fibrous membrane serves as a protective covering for bones. It contains nerves and blood vessels that nourish the bone, facilitating growth and repair. Beneath the periosteum lies the compact bone, a dense and hard layer that provides strength and support. This part of the bone is what gives it its rigidity and ability to bear weight. Compact bone is organized into tightly packed structures called osteons, which are cylindrical units that run parallel to the bone's long axis.

Inside the compact bone is the spongy bone, also known as cancellous bone. Unlike the dense compact bone, spongy bone has a porous, honeycomb-like structure. This design makes it lighter and provides space for bone marrow. Spongy bone is highly vascularized, meaning it has a rich supply of blood vessels, which is essential for producing blood cells.

At the core of many bones lies the bone marrow. There are two types of bone marrow: red and yellow. Red bone marrow is responsible for producing red blood cells, white blood cells, and platelets. It is found mainly in flat bones such as the pelvis, sternum, and ribs. Yellow bone marrow, on the other hand, consists primarily of fat cells and is found in the long bones of adults. Over time, red bone marrow can convert to yellow marrow, reflecting a shift in the body's needs as we age.

Bones also have an inner lining called the endosteum, which lines the internal marrow cavity. This thin membrane plays a crucial role in bone growth and remodeling. It contains osteoblasts, cells responsible for forming new bone, and osteoclasts, cells that break down old bone. This balance between formation and resorption is essential for maintaining bone density and strength.

The functions of bones extend beyond mere support and structure. They protect our vital organs; the skull encases the brain, the rib cage shields the heart and lungs, and the vertebrae safeguard the spinal cord. Bones also serve as reservoirs for minerals, particularly calcium and phosphorus. These minerals are essential for various bodily functions, including nerve transmission and muscle contraction. When the body needs these minerals, it can draw from the bone's stores, highlighting the importance of maintaining bone health.

Bone remodeling is a continuous process where old bone tissue is replaced by new tissue. This process is vital for repairing microdamages and ensuring bone strength. Osteoblasts and osteoclasts are the cells at the forefront of this activity. Osteoblasts are responsible for forming new bone by secreting a matrix that becomes mineralized. Conversely, osteoclasts break down old bone by dissolving minerals and resorbing the bone matrix. This dynamic balance between osteoblasts and osteoclasts is crucial for bone health.

As we age, the balance between bone formation and resorption can shift. In younger individuals, bone formation outpaces resorption, leading to growth and increased bone density. However, with advancing age, this balance often tips in favor of resorption, resulting in a gradual loss of bone density. This age-related bone loss can increase the risk of fractures and other bone-related issues.

Familiarizing yourself with key bone health terminology can help you better understand and manage your bone health. Bone mineral density (BMD) measures the number of minerals in your bones, indicating their strength and density. A higher BMD generally means stronger bones, while a lower BMD can signal a risk for conditions like osteoporosis. Peak bone mass refers to the maximum bone density and strength you achieve, usually in your late twenties. Maintaining this peak bone mass through proper nutrition, exercise, and lifestyle choices is crucial for long-term bone health.

Understanding the anatomy and functions of bones, along with the processes of bone remodeling, provides a solid foundation for the strategies and recommendations that will follow in this book. By grasping these concepts, you will be better equipped to take proactive steps in maintaining and improving your bone health, ensuring a more active and fulfilling life as you age.

1.2 OSTEOPOROSIS AND OSTEOPENIA: DIFFERENCES AND DIAGNOSES

Osteoporosis and osteopenia are two conditions that signify varying degrees of bone loss, but they differ significantly in severity and implications. Osteoporosis is characterized by severe bone loss, making bones weak and brittle. This condition increases the likelihood of fractures from minor incidents such as a simple fall, or even a cough or sneeze. On the other hand, osteopenia represents a milder form of bone loss. While the bones are weaker than normal, they are not as fragile as in osteoporosis. However, without proper management, osteopenia can progress to osteoporosis, increasing the risk of severe complications.

Several risk factors contribute to the development of osteoporosis and osteopenia. Age and gender play a significant role, with postmenopausal women being at a higher risk due to the decline in estrogen levels, which is crucial for bone density maintenance. Family history also influences the likelihood of developing these conditions. If your parents or siblings have experienced osteoporosis or fractures, your risk increases. Lifestyle factors such as smoking and excessive alcohol consumption further exacerbate the risk. Smoking interferes with the body's ability to absorb calcium, while alcohol affects bone formation and increases the risk of falls due to impaired balance and coordination.

The diagnostic process for osteoporosis and osteopenia typically involves a bone density test known as a dual-energy X-ray absorptiometry (DEXA) scan. This scan measures bone mineral density (BMD) and compares it to the optimal peak bone density of a healthy young adult. The results are given as T-scores and Z-scores. A T-score of -1.0 or above is considered normal, between -1.0 and -2.5 indicates osteopenia, and -2.5 or below signifies osteoporosis. The Z-score compares your bone density to what is expected for someone of your age, sex, and size. While less commonly used for diagnosis, it can provide additional context, especially for younger individuals or those with secondary causes of bone loss.

Receiving a diagnosis of osteoporosis or osteopenia brings significant implications for daily life and long-term health. One of the most immediate concerns is the increased risk of fractures. For seniors, a fracture can lead to a cascade of health issues, including decreased mobility, loss of independence, and a diminished quality of life. For example, hip fractures often require surgery and extensive rehabilitation, and they can be life-threatening. The potential impact on mobility cannot be overstated. Reduced bone density means that even minor falls can result in serious injuries, making it crucial to adopt preventive measures to minimize fall risks, such as using assistive devices, ensuring adequate lighting in the home, and removing tripping hazards.

Beyond the physical implications, there are also psychological and emotional effects to consider. The fear of falling and the potential for fractures can lead to a more sedentary lifestyle, which further exacerbates bone loss and decreases muscle strength. This cycle can create a sense of helplessness and anxiety, impacting overall mental well-being. Understanding these implications underscores the importance of early diagnosis and proactive management of bone health.

In managing osteoporosis or osteopenia, knowledge is a powerful tool. By understanding the risk factors, you can take proactive steps to mitigate them. For instance, if you have a family history of osteoporosis, it becomes even more critical to adopt a bone-healthy lifestyle early on. This includes engaging in regular weight-bearing and muscle-strengthening exercises, consuming a diet rich in calcium and vitamin D, and avoiding smoking and excessive alcohol. Moreover, regular check-ups and bone density tests can help monitor your bone health and detect any changes early, allowing for timely intervention.

In the next sections of this book, we will explore various strategies to manage and improve bone health. These include detailed exercise routines tailored for different fitness levels, nutritional guidance to ensure you are getting the necessary nutrients for bone strength, and information on supplements that can support bone health. We will also delve into lifestyle changes that can make a significant difference and discuss medical options available for managing osteoporosis and osteopenia. By integrating these strategies into your daily life, you can take control of your bone health and reduce the risks associated with these conditions.

Understanding osteoporosis and osteopenia is the first step towards managing them effectively. By recognizing the differences between these conditions and being aware of the risk factors, you are better equipped to take proactive measures. The diagnostic process, while straightforward, provides crucial information that guides treatment and management strategies. The implications of a diagnosis highlight the importance of maintaining bone health, not just for physical well-being, but also for mental and emotional health. As we continue through this book, you will gain the knowledge and tools to improve your bone health, ensuring a more active, independent, and fulfilling life.

1.3 ARTHRITIS: TYPES, SYMPTOMS, AND BONE HEALTH IMPACT

Arthritis, a common condition among seniors, manifests in various forms, each affecting the joints and bones differently. Understanding the types of arthritis and their impact on bone health is crucial for effective management and improving the quality of life. The most prevalent forms of arthritis affecting seniors include osteoarthritis, rheumatoid arthritis, and psoriatic arthritis. Each type has distinct characteristics and implications for bone health.

Osteoarthritis is the most common form of arthritis, often referred to as a wear-and-tear disease. It occurs when the protective cartilage that cushions the ends of your bones wears down over time. This degeneration leads to bones rubbing against each other, causing pain, swelling, and reduced joint mobility. Osteoarthritis commonly affects the knees, hips, and hands, making everyday activities like walking, climbing stairs, and gripping objects challenging. The damage to the joints can result in bone spurs, further contributing to pain and stiffness.

Rheumatoid arthritis, an autoimmune disease, occurs when the immune system mistakenly attacks the body's tissues, specifically the synovium—the lining of the membranes that surround the joints. This leads to inflammation, which can eventually result in bone erosion and joint deformity. Unlike osteoarthritis, rheumatoid arthritis affects more than just the joints. It can also damage other body systems, including the skin, eyes, lungs, heart, and blood vessels. This systemic nature of rheumatoid arthritis means that its impact on bone health is both direct and indirect, leading to increased risk of osteoporosis and fractures.

Psoriatic arthritis affects some individuals who have psoriasis, a condition characterized by red patches of skin topped with silvery scales. This type of arthritis involves joint pain, stiffness, and swelling, which can range from mild to severe. Psoriatic arthritis can affect any part of the body, including the fingertips and spine, and its symptoms can flare up and subside unpredictably. The inflammation associated with psoriatic arthritis can lead to significant joint damage and an increased risk of bone loss.

Arthritis symptoms can vary depending on the type and severity of the condition. Common symptoms include joint pain and stiffness, which can be particularly pronounced in the morning or after periods of inactivity. Swelling and inflammation are also frequent, as the body's immune response targets the affected joints. This swelling can cause tenderness and warmth around the joints, making movement painful. Reduced range of motion is another common symptom, as the joints become less flexible and more difficult to move. This limitation can interfere with daily activities and diminish the overall quality of life.

The impact of arthritis on bone health extends beyond joint damage. Chronic inflammation associated with rheumatoid and psoriatic arthritis can accelerate the process of bone resorption, leading to decreased bone density and increased risk of fractures. Joint damage and bone erosion are common, particularly in rheumatoid arthritis, where the immune system's attack on the synovium leads to the destruction of cartilage and bone within the joint. This damage can result in joint deformities and significant functional impairments. Additionally, arthritis can increase the risk of falls due to joint instability and reduced mobility, further exacerbating the risk of fractures.

Managing arthritis involves a multifaceted approach that includes medications, physical therapy, chiropractic adjustments, and dietary adjustments. Medications such as non-steroidal anti-inflammatory drugs (NSAIDs) can help reduce pain and inflammation, making it easier to move and perform daily activities. Disease-modifying antirheumatic drugs (DMARDs) are often prescribed for rheumatoid arthritis to slow the progression of the disease and prevent joint damage. Biologic agents, a newer class of DMARDs, target specific components of the immune system to reduce inflammation and halt disease progression.

Physical therapy plays a crucial role in managing arthritis by improving joint function and mobility. A physical therapist can design a personalized exercise program that includes range-of-motion exercises, strengthening exercises, and aerobic activities. These exercises help maintain joint flexibility, build muscle strength, and improve overall physical fitness. Regular physical activity can also help manage weight, reducing the stress on weight bearing joints and alleviating some of the symptoms of arthritis.

Chiropractic adjustments can provide relief for individuals with arthritis by improving joint mobility and reducing pain. Chiropractors use hands-on techniques to manipulate the spine and other joints, aiming to restore proper alignment and function. These adjustments can help reduce joint inflammation and improve range of motion, contributing to better overall joint health. However, it's helpful to consult a healthcare provider before starting chiropractic treatment to ensure it's appropriate for your specific condition.

Dietary adjustments can also play a significant role in managing arthritis. Consuming a balanced diet rich in anti-inflammatory foods, such as fruits, vegetables, whole grains, and omega-3 fatty acids, can help reduce inflammation and support overall health. Foods high in antioxidants, such as berries and leafy greens, can help combat oxidative stress, which contributes to inflammation and joint damage. Additionally, maintaining a healthy weight through proper nutrition can reduce the burden on weight-bearing joints, alleviating some of the symptoms of arthritis.

Managing arthritis requires a comprehensive approach that addresses the condition's various aspects. By understanding the different types of arthritis, recognizing the symptoms, and implementing effective management strategies, you can take control of your condition and improve your bone health. This holistic approach will help you maintain better joint function, reduce pain, and enhance your overall quality of life.

1.4 THE SCIENCE BEHIND BONE DENSITY

Bone density is a pivotal aspect of overall bone health. It refers to the amount of mineral content, primarily calcium and phosphate, within a specific volume of bone, measured in grams per square centimeter (g/cm^2). This measurement provides a clear indicator of bone strength and resilience against fractures. Higher bone density signifies stronger bones capable of withstanding stress, while lower bone density indicates weaker bones prone to breaks and fractures. Understanding bone density is crucial because it not only determines the robustness of your skeletal system but also serves as a predictor for conditions like osteoporosis and osteopenia.

Several factors influence bone density, with genetics playing a significant role. If your parents or grandparents had a history of osteoporosis, you might be predisposed to lower bone density. This genetic link means that despite your best efforts, some aspects of bone health are inherited. However, genetics is just one piece of the puzzle. Hormonal changes, particularly those occurring during menopause, significantly impact bone density. Estrogen, a hormone that helps maintain bone density, decreases sharply during menopause, leading to an increased rate of bone resorption and a subsequent decline in bone density.

Nutrition is another critical factor affecting bone density. Calcium and vitamin D are essential nutrients for maintaining strong bones. Calcium provides the building blocks for bone tissue, while vitamin D enhances the absorption of calcium from the diet. A deficiency in either nutrient can lead to weakened bones and increased risk of fractures. Consuming a balanced diet rich in these nutrients can help maintain bone density. Foods such as dairy products, leafy green vegetables, and fortified cereals are excellent sources of calcium. Sunlight exposure and foods like fatty fish and fortified milk can help provide adequate vitamin D.

Lifestyle choices have a profound impact on bone density. Physical activity, particularly weight-bearing and resistance exercises, stimulates bone formation and increases bone density. Activities like walking, jogging, dancing, and lifting weights apply stress to the bones, prompting them to become denser and stronger. In contrast, a sedentary lifestyle can lead to bone loss and decreased bone density. Smoking and alcohol consumption are detrimental to bone health. Smoking interferes with the absorption of calcium, while excessive alcohol consumption affects bone formation and increases the risk of falls, which can lead to fractures.

There are several strategies to improve and maintain bone density. Nutritional supplements can play a crucial role, especially if dietary intake is insufficient. Calcium and vitamin D supplements are commonly recommended to support bone health. However, it's essential to consult a healthcare provider before starting any supplementation to determine the appropriate dosage and avoid potential side effects. Regular exercise routines that include weight-bearing and resistance exercises are vital for maintaining bone density. Aim for at least 30 minutes of physical activity most days of the week. Incorporate exercises that target different muscle groups and use various forms of resistance, such as free weights, resistance bands, or body-weight exercises.

Medication options are available for individuals at high risk of fractures or those diagnosed with osteoporosis. Bisphosphonates are a class of drugs commonly prescribed to slow down bone resorption, allowing the bone formation process to catch up, thereby increasing bone density. These medications are usually taken orally or through intravenous infusion, depending on the specific drug and patient needs. Another option is hormone replacement therapy (HRT), which can be effective for post-menopausal women by supplementing estrogen levels. However, HRT may have side effects and is not suitable for everyone, so it should be discussed thoroughly with a healthcare provider.

Improving and maintaining bone density requires a multifaceted approach. A combination of proper nutrition, regular physical activity, and, when necessary, medication can help ensure bones remain strong and healthy. It's also essential to avoid smoking and limit alcohol consumption, as these habits can undermine efforts to maintain bone density. Regular check-ups and bone density tests can help monitor progress and make necessary adjustments to your bone health strategy.

Understanding the science behind bone density empowers you to take proactive steps in maintaining your bone health. By recognizing the factors that influence bone density and adopting strategies to improve it, you can reduce the risk of fractures and enjoy a more active and independent life. The importance of bone density extends beyond just physical health; it also impacts overall wellbeing and quality of life. Taking care of your bones now will pay dividends in the years to come, allowing you to continue doing the things you love without the fear of fractures or bone-related complications.

2

MEDICAL OPTIONS AND EXPLANATIONS

When I reflect on my years of practice, I recall a patient named George, who was a vibrant 68-year-old. He led an active life but was suddenly alarmed by a simple fall that resulted in a wrist fracture. Confused and concerned, George sought answers. It was a bone density scan that revealed the underlying issue—osteoporosis. This pivotal moment in his life underscores the importance of understanding and utilizing medical options to manage bone health effectively.

2.1 BONE DENSITY SCANS: WHAT THEY REVEAL

Bone density scans are indispensable tools in diagnosing and managing bone health conditions such as osteoporosis and osteopenia. These scans are crucial because they allow for the early detection of bone density issues, enabling timely intervention and treatment. Early detection is paramount; it helps prevent fractures and other complications that can arise from weakened bones. Moreover, these scans serve as valuable tools for monitoring changes in bone density over time, allowing healthcare providers to assess the effectiveness of treatments and make necessary adjustments.

Several types of bone density scans are used to measure bone mineral density (BMD). The most common and widely recognized method is the Dual-energy X-ray Absorptiometry, or DEXA scan. This scan uses a small dose of ionizing radiation to measure bone loss, making it a quick and noninvasive procedure. DEXA scans are typically performed on the lower spine and hips, and in some cases, the whole body or peripheral areas like the forearm may be scanned. Another method is Peripheral Quantitative Computed Tomography (pQCT), which provides a three-dimensional assessment of bone density and strength. While less common than DEXA, pQCT offers detailed insights into bone structure and is particularly useful in research settings.

Undergoing a bone density scan is a straightforward process. Before the scan, you may be advised to avoid taking calcium supplements for at least 24 hours. This precaution ensures that the scan results are accurate and not influenced by recent calcium intake. The procedure itself is quick, typically taking between 10 and 30 minutes. During the scan, you will lie on a padded table while a scanning arm passes over your body. The scan is painless and involves minimal discomfort, similar to undergoing a standard X-ray. You can expect to remain still during the procedure to ensure clear and precise images.

Understanding the results of a bone density scan is crucial for making informed decisions about your bone health. The results are typically reported as T-scores and Z-scores. A T-score compares your bone density to that of a healthy young adult of the same gender. A T-score of -1.0 or above is considered normal, indicating healthy bone density. A T-score between -1.0 and -2.5 indicates osteopenia, a condition where bone density is below normal but not low enough to be classified as osteoporosis. A T-score of -2.5 or lower signifies osteoporosis, indicating a significant risk of fractures and the need for medical intervention.

In addition to T-scores, bone density scans also provide Z-scores. A Z-score compares your bone density to the average bone density of people your age, gender, and size. While Z-scores are less commonly used for diagnosing osteoporosis, they can provide valuable context, especially for younger individuals or those with secondary causes of bone loss. A Z-score of -2.0 or lower suggests that your bone density is significantly below the expected range for your age, potentially indicating underlying health issues that need further investigation.

Bone density scans are a cornerstone in the diagnosis and management of bone health conditions. They offer a clear and objective measure of bone strength, enabling early detection of osteoporosis and osteopenia. By understanding the types of scans available, the procedure involved, and how to interpret the results, you can take proactive steps to maintain and improve your bone health. Regular bone density scans, combined with a holistic approach to bone health, can significantly reduce the risk of fractures and ensure a better quality of life as you age.

Interactive Element: Preparing for Your Bone Density Scan

To ensure the most accurate results from your bone density scan, consider the following checklist:

- Avoid taking calcium supplements 24 hours before the scan.
- Wear loose, comfortable clothing without metal zippers or buttons.

- Inform the technician if you have recently had any other medical procedures involving contrast material.
- Bring a list of your current medications and supplements.
- Arrive at the appointment a few minutes early to complete any necessary paperwork.

By following these simple steps, you can help ensure that your bone density scan provides the most accurate and useful information for managing your bone health.

2.2 PRESCRIPTION MEDICATIONS: BENEFITS AND SIDE EFFECTS

When managing bone health, especially conditions like osteoporosis and arthritis, prescription medications play a critical role. These medications are designed to either slow down bone loss or stimulate bone formation, providing a range of benefits for those affected. Among the most commonly prescribed drugs for bone health are bisphosphonates, selective estrogen receptor modulators (SERMs), and parathyroid hormone (PTH) analogs.

Bisphosphonates, such as Alendronate and Risedronate, are often the first line of defense in treating osteoporosis. These medications work by inhibiting the activity of osteoclasts, the cells responsible for breaking down bone tissue. By reducing bone resorption, bisphosphonates help to maintain or increase bone density, thereby reducing the risk of fractures. Selective estrogen receptor modulators (SERMs), on the other hand, mimic the effects of estrogen on bone tissue. Estrogen is crucial for maintaining bone density, and SERMs like Raloxifene can help preserve bone mass in postmenopausal women. Parathyroid hormone (PTH) analogs, such as Teriparatide, are another option. These medications stimulate bone formation by increasing the activity of osteoblasts, the cells responsible for building new bone tissue.

The benefits of these medications are significant. Increased bone density is perhaps the most immediate and measurable advantage. By preserving or enhancing bone mass, these drugs reduce the risk of fractures, which is a primary concern for individuals with osteoporosis. For those suffering from arthritis, certain medications can also provide pain relief, improving overall quality of life. The ability to manage pain effectively allows individuals to maintain a more active lifestyle, which in turn supports bone health.

However, like all medications, these drugs come with potential side effects. Bisphosphonates, while effective, can cause gastrointestinal issues such as nausea, heartburn, and esophageal irritation. In rare cases, long-term use of bisphosphonates has been linked to osteonecrosis of the jaw, a condition where the jawbone begins to weaken and die. This risk underscores the importance of regular dental check-ups for anyone taking these medications. SERMs, while beneficial for bone density, can cause hot flashes, especially in postmenopausal women. These hot flashes can be uncomfortable and may affect daily activities. Parathyroid hormone analogs, although effective in stimulating bone formation, can result in side effects like leg cramps and dizziness, making it crucial to discuss any new symptoms with your healthcare provider.

Managing these side effects involves a combination of strategies. Taking bisphosphonates with food or water can help minimize gastrointestinal discomfort. It is also advisable to remain upright for at least 30 minutes after taking the medication to prevent esophageal irritation. Regular dental check-ups are essential for monitoring jaw health, especially for those on long-term bisphosphonate therapy. For individuals experiencing hot flashes due to SERMs, lifestyle adjustments such as dressing in layers, keeping the environment cool, and avoiding triggers like spicy foods and caffeine can provide relief. If side effects become severe or unmanageable, consulting with a healthcare provider is crucial. They may adjust the dosage or suggest alternative medications that offer similar benefits with fewer adverse effects.

Parathyroid hormone analogs require careful monitoring due to their potential side effects. If you experience leg cramps or dizziness, it's essential to report these symptoms to your healthcare provider promptly. They may recommend adjustments to your medication regimen or suggest complementary therapies to alleviate these issues. Additionally, incorporating a balanced diet rich in calcium and vitamin D can support the effectiveness of these medications and contribute to overall bone health. Regular physical activity, tailored to your abilities and limitations, can also enhance the benefits of medication by promoting bone strength and flexibility.

Understanding the range of prescription medications available for bone health, along with their benefits and potential side effects, empowers you to make informed decisions about your treatment plan. By working closely with your healthcare provider and adopting strategies to manage side effects, you can optimize your bone health and reduce the risk of fractures and other complications.

2.3 INTERPRETING YOUR BONE HEALTH REPORT

Your bone health report is a crucial document that provides a comprehensive overview of your bone density and fracture risk. Understanding this report will enable you to make informed decisions about your bone health management. The report typically begins with bone density results, presented as T-scores and Z-scores. T-scores compare your bone density to that of a healthy young adult. This comparison helps determine whether your bone density falls within the normal range, indicates osteopenia, or suggests osteoporosis. A T-score of -1.0 or above is considered normal, while a score between -1.0 and -2.5 points to osteopenia. A T-score of -2.5 or lower signifies osteoporosis, signaling a higher risk for fractures and the need for medical intervention.

Z-scores, on the other hand, compare your bone density to the average bone density of people your age, gender, and size. While less commonly used for diagnosing osteoporosis, Z-scores offer valuable context, especially for younger individuals or those with secondary causes of bone loss. A Z-score of -2.0 or lower suggests that your bone density is significantly below the expected range for your demographic, potentially indicating underlying health issues that require further investigation. Understanding these scores is essential for grasping the state of your bone health.

Another critical component of your bone health report is the fracture risk assessment. This assessment estimates your likelihood of experiencing a fracture within the next ten years. Factors such as age, gender, family history, and previous fractures are considered in this assessment. The Fracture Risk Assessment Tool (FRAX) is often used to calculate this risk. A high fracture risk means you need to take immediate steps to strengthen your bones and minimize fall risks. This might include lifestyle changes, medications, or both.

The report also includes recommended follow-up actions. These recommendations are based on your bone density results and fracture risk assessment. If your scores indicate osteopenia or osteoporosis, your healthcare provider may suggest specific medications to slow bone loss or stimulate bone formation. They might also recommend lifestyle changes such as incorporating weight-bearing exercises, ensuring adequate calcium and vitamin

D intake, and avoiding smoking and excessive alcohol consumption. Regular follow-up scans may be advised to monitor your bone density over time and assess the effectiveness of any treatments you are undergoing.

Interpreting your bone health report requires a thorough understanding of the scores and their implications. A normal T-score indicates healthy bone density, while a T-score in the osteopenia range suggests a need for preventive measures to avoid progression to osteoporosis. If your T-score falls within the osteoporosis range, immediate action is necessary to reduce fracture risk. Z-scores provide additional context, especially if they are significantly below the expected range for your age group. These scores can help identify potential underlying conditions affecting your bone health.

The significance of the findings in your bone health report cannot be overstated. High fracture risk means you are more likely to experience fractures, which can severely impact your mobility and quality of life. Understanding this risk allows you to take proactive steps to strengthen your bones and reduce the likelihood of fractures. Follow-up scans are crucial for monitoring changes in your bone density and adjusting your treatment plan as needed. Regular monitoring helps ensure that any interventions are effective and allows for timely adjustments.

Once you receive your bone health report, discussing the results with your healthcare provider is essential. They can help you understand the implications of your scores and recommend appropriate treatments or lifestyle changes. Implementing these recommendations is crucial for improving your bone health. This might involve starting a new medication, adjusting your diet to include more bone-healthy nutrients, or beginning a regular exercise routine focused on weight-bearing and resistance exercises.

Your healthcare provider can also help you set realistic goals and create a plan to achieve them.

Taking action after receiving your bone health report is vital for maintaining and improving your bone health. Discussing the results with your healthcare provider will give you a clear understanding of your bone density and fracture risk. Implementing recommended lifestyle changes, such as incorporating weight-bearing exercises and ensuring adequate calcium and vitamin D intake, can significantly improve your bone health. Considering medication options, if advised, can also help slow bone loss and stimulate bone formation, reducing your risk of fractures and enhancing your quality of life.

2.4 DISCUSSING TREATMENT PLANS WITH YOUR DOCTOR

When preparing for your appointment with your healthcare provider, it's crucial to come well-prepared. Start by compiling a list of all current medications and supplements you are taking. This list should include prescription drugs, over-the-counter medicines, vitamins, and herbal supplements. Having this comprehensive list ensures that your doctor has a complete picture of your health and can make informed decisions about your treatment plan. Additionally, prepare a set of questions you want to ask about your treatment options. Consider asking about the benefits and risks of each potential treatment, how long you might need to take the medication, and what side effects to watch for.

Setting clear treatment goals is another essential step in your discussion with your healthcare provider. These goals will guide your treatment plan and help you and your doctor measure progress. One primary goal should be preventing fractures, as these can severely impact your mobility and quality of life.

Improving bone density is another critical objective, as stronger bones mean a lower risk of fractures. Managing symptoms of arthritis, such as pain and stiffness, can also be a vital goal if you have this condition. By clearly outlining your goals, you provide a focus for your treatment plan, making it easier to track improvements and make necessary adjustments.

Reviewing potential treatments with your doctor involves a thorough evaluation of all available options. Your doctor may present various medications, lifestyle changes, and non-pharmaceutical interventions. Comparing these options involves looking at the effectiveness, potential side effects, and your personal preferences. Medications might offer quick relief and significant improvements in bone density, but they may come with side effects that require careful management. On the other hand, lifestyle changes, such as regular exercise and dietary adjustments, might take longer to show results but come with fewer risks. Non-pharmaceutical interventions, like physical therapy or acupuncture, can also be effective and may align better with your preferences for natural treatment options.

During your discussion, it's vital to address any concerns or preferences you have regarding your treatment plan. Open communication with your healthcare provider ensures that your treatment aligns with your values and lifestyle. For instance, if you have concerns about the side effects of a particular medication, discuss these openly. Your doctor can provide further instructions and may suggest alternative treatments that carry fewer risks. If you prefer natural treatment options, such as dietary changes and exercise, express this preference. Your doctor can help you develop a treatment plan that incorporates these elements while still effectively managing your bone health.

Addressing your concerns also means discussing any fears you might have about starting a new treatment. Fear of side effects is common and understandable. Your doctor can provide strategies for managing these side effects, such as taking medications with food or water to minimize gastrointestinal discomfort. Regular dental check-ups might be recommended if you're taking medications that affect jaw health. If side effects become too severe, your doctor can adjust the dosage or suggest alternative medications. By discussing these concerns, you can feel more confident and comfortable with your treatment plan.

Exploring natural treatment options is another important aspect of your discussion with your healthcare provider. Many individuals prefer to manage their bone health through diet, exercise, and other non-pharmaceutical methods. If this is your preference, let your doctor know. They can help you identify the most effective natural treatments and ensure that these methods are safe and beneficial for your specific condition. For example, your doctor might recommend a diet rich in calcium and vitamin D to support bone health, along with weight-bearing exercises to strengthen your bones. They might also suggest physical therapy to improve mobility and reduce pain.

In preparing for your appointment, consider writing down your treatment goals and any questions or concerns you have. Bringing this written list to your appointment can help ensure that you cover all important topics and make the most of your time with your healthcare provider. Remember that your doctor is there to help you navigate your bone health journey, and open, honest communication is key to developing an effective treatment plan that meets your needs.

2.5 NON-PHARMACEUTICAL INTERVENTIONS FOR BONE HEALTH

Lifestyle changes play a pivotal role in managing bone health. While medications can offer significant benefits, integrating non-pharmaceutical interventions into your daily routine can substantially improve bone density and overall well-being. Regular weight-bearing exercises are one of the most effective ways to maintain and enhance bone health. Activities such as walking, jogging, and dancing apply stress to your bones, prompting them to become denser and stronger. Incorporating these exercises into your daily routine can help prevent bone loss and reduce the risk of fractures. Alongside physical activity, a balanced diet rich in calcium and vitamin D is crucial. Calcium is the primary building block of bone tissue, while vitamin D enhances calcium absorption, ensuring that your bones receive the nutrients they need to remain robust. Foods such as dairy products, leafy greens, and fortified cereals are excellent sources of calcium, while sunlight exposure and fatty fish can help you obtain sufficient vitamin D.

Beyond dietary and exercise modifications, several alternative therapies can support bone health. Physical therapy is a valuable non-drug intervention that focuses on improving mobility, strength, and balance. A physical therapist can design a personalized exercise program tailored to your specific needs, including range-of-motion exercises, strengthening routines, and balance training. These exercises not only enhance bone density but also improve muscle strength and coordination, reducing the risk of falls. Additionally, physical therapy can address any existing mobility issues, helping you maintain an active and independent lifestyle.

Acupuncture is another alternative therapy that can be beneficial for bone health, particularly in managing pain associated with osteoporosis and arthritis. This ancient practice involves inserting thin needles into specific points on the body to stimulate the nervous system and promote natural pain relief. Acupuncture can help reduce inflammation, alleviate pain, and improve overall well-being. Many individuals find that regular acupuncture sessions provide significant relief from chronic pain, allowing them to engage more fully in physical activities that support bone health. While scientific evidence on acupuncture's efficacy is still evolving, many seniors report positive outcomes from integrating this therapy into their bone health management plan.

Yoga is an excellent practice for enhancing balance, flexibility, and overall bone health. Yoga poses, or asanas, involve weight-bearing movements that can strengthen bones and improve joint function. Practices such as standing poses, balancing poses, and gentle twists can help increase bone density while enhancing flexibility and muscle strength. Yoga also promotes mindfulness and relaxation, reducing stress levels that can negatively impact bone health. Incorporating yoga into your routine a few times a week can provide both physical and mental benefits, supporting a holistic approach to bone health.

Chiropractic adjustments can also play a role in improving bone health by enhancing alignment and mobility. Chiropractors use hands-on techniques to manipulate the spine and other joints, aiming to restore proper alignment and function. These adjustments can help reduce joint inflammation, improve range of motion, and alleviate pain. For individuals with osteoporosis or arthritis, regular chiropractic care can complement other treatments by addressing musculoskeletal issues and promoting overall well-being. It's essential to consult a healthcare provider before starting chiropractic treatment to ensure it's appropriate for your specific condition.

Integrating these non-pharmaceutical interventions into your bone health management plan can provide substantial benefits. Regular weight-bearing exercises, a balanced diet rich in calcium and vitamin D, and alternative therapies such as physical therapy, acupuncture, yoga, and chiropractic adjustments all contribute to stronger bones and improved overall health. By adopting a holistic approach to bone health, you can reduce your reliance on medications, minimize side effects, and enjoy a more active and fulfilling life.

In the next chapter, we will delve into nutritional guidance, exploring how a well-balanced diet can further support bone health and complement the lifestyle changes and alternative therapies discussed here.

3

NUTRITIONAL GUIDANCE FOR BONE HEALTH

Years ago, I met Helen, a lively 74-year-old who loved gardening and playing with her grandchildren. She came to me puzzled about why she was experiencing frequent fractures despite her active lifestyle. After a detailed conversation, it became clear that her diet was lacking in one crucial element—calcium. Helen's story underscores the importance of understanding calcium's role in bone health, particularly for seniors.

3.1 UNDERSTANDING CALCIUM AND ITS ROLE IN BONE HEALTH

Calcium is an indispensable mineral for maintaining strong and healthy bones. It is the most abundant mineral in the human body, with 99% of it stored in our bones and teeth. Calcium plays a vital role in providing structural support and maintaining bone mass. Bones are not static; they are living tissues that constantly undergo remodeling, a process where old bone is broken down and new bone is formed. Calcium is essential for this process, ensuring that bones remain dense and resilient. Without adequate calcium, the body starts to withdraw calcium from bones, making them weak and more susceptible to fractures.

Beyond its role in bone composition, calcium is crucial for several physiological functions. It aids in muscle function, allowing muscles to contract and relax properly. This is particularly important for seniors, as muscle function can impact mobility and balance, reducing the risk of falls. Calcium also plays a key role in nerve signaling, facilitating communication between the brain and other parts of the body. This communication is essential for coordinating movements and ensuring the proper functioning of various bodily systems. Additionally, calcium helps in blood clotting and maintaining a normal heartbeat, further highlighting its multifaceted importance in overall health.

For seniors, meeting daily calcium requirements is vital for maintaining bone density and preventing osteoporosis. The recommended daily allowance (RDA) for calcium varies by age and gender. Women aged 51 and older need 1,200 milligrams of calcium per day, while men aged 51 to 70 require 1,000 milligrams daily. After age 70, the requirement for men increases to 1,200 milligrams. These recommendations consider the natural decline in calcium absorption and bone density that occurs with age. Ensuring you meet these daily requirements is crucial for maintaining strong bones and reducing the risk of fractures.

Incorporating calcium-rich foods into your diet is an effective way to meet these requirements. Dairy products are among the best sources of calcium. Milk, cheese, and yogurt are not only rich in calcium but also provide other essential nutrients like protein and vitamin D. For example, a cup of milk contains about 300 milligrams of calcium, while an ounce of cheese can provide roughly 200 milligrams. Yogurt is another excellent option, with a cup offering up to 450 milligrams of calcium.

Leafy green vegetables are also valuable sources of calcium. Kale, collard greens, and broccoli are particularly high in calcium, with a cup of cooked collard greens providing about 268 milligrams. Fortified foods can further enhance your calcium intake. Many cereals, orange juices, and plant-based milks are fortified with calcium, offering a convenient way to boost your daily intake.

However, simply consuming calcium-rich foods is not enough; the body must also efficiently absorb this calcium. Several factors can influence calcium absorption. Vitamin D plays a crucial role in this process. It enhances calcium absorption in the intestines, ensuring that the calcium you consume is effectively utilized by the body. Without sufficient vitamin D, even a calcium-rich diet may not be enough to maintain bone health. Foods like fatty fish, fortified milk, and egg yolks are good sources of vitamin D. Sunlight exposure also helps the body produce vitamin D, making outdoor activities beneficial for both bone health and overall well-being.

Certain compounds in foods can impact calcium absorption. Oxalates and phytates, found in foods like spinach, rhubarb, and whole grains, can bind to calcium and reduce its absorption. While these foods are nutritious and should not be avoided, it is essential to balance your diet to ensure adequate calcium intake. For instance, consuming calcium-rich foods with vitamin D sources can enhance absorption, while spreading your calcium intake throughout the day can prevent the body from becoming overwhelmed, allowing for more efficient utilization.

Interactive Element: Track Your Calcium Intake

To ensure you are meeting your daily calcium requirements, consider keeping a food diary for a week. Note down all the foods you eat and their calcium content. This practice can help you identify any gaps in your diet and make necessary adjustments. Here is a simple checklist to get you started:

- Milk: 1 cup (300 mg)
- Cheese: 1 ounce (200 mg)
- Yogurt: 1 cup (450 mg)
- Kale: 1 cup cooked (100 mg)
- Fortified orange juice: 1 cup (350 mg)

By tracking your intake, you can ensure you are consuming enough calcium to support your bone health, making adjustments as needed to maintain strong and resilient bones.

3.2 VITAMIN D: THE SUNSHINE VITAMIN'S ROLE IN BONE DENSITY

Vitamin D, often called the "sunshine vitamin," plays a crucial role in maintaining bone health. It facilitates the absorption of calcium from the gut into the bloodstream, making sure that the calcium you consume is effectively utilized by your body. Without sufficient vitamin D, calcium absorption can drop significantly, leading to weaker bones. Additionally, vitamin D helps modulate bone remodeling, the process where old bone is broken down and new bone is formed. This balance is essential for maintaining bone density and strength, particularly as we age.

There are several ways to obtain sufficient vitamin D. The most natural method is through sunlight exposure. When your skin is exposed to sunlight, it synthesizes vitamin D. Aim for about 10 to 30 minutes of midday sunlight several times a week, depending on your skin type and the strength of the sun. However, it's essential to balance sun exposure with skin cancer risk, so always use sunscreen after the initial exposure period. Dietary sources of vitamin D are also valuable. Fatty fish like salmon, mackerel, and trout are excellent sources. One serving of salmon can provide up to 570 international units (IU) of vitamin D. Egg yolks and fortified foods like milk, orange juice, and cereals can also help you meet your daily vitamin D needs.

The recommended daily allowance (RDA) for vitamin D varies by age and gender. For adults up to age 70, the RDA is 600 IU per day. For those over 70, the RDA increases to 800 IU daily to account for the decreased efficiency in synthesizing vitamin D from sunlight. If you have limited sun exposure, perhaps due to living in northern latitudes or spending much of your time indoors, you might need to rely more on dietary sources and supplements. It's crucial to consult your healthcare provider to determine the appropriate dosage for your specific needs, especially since excessive vitamin D can lead to toxicity and other health issues.

Vitamin D deficiency can have significant consequences for your bone health. Common symptoms include fatigue, bone pain, and muscle weakness. These symptoms can be subtle and easily overlooked, but they indicate that your body is not getting enough vitamin D to support its functions. A prolonged deficiency can lead to more severe conditions like osteomalacia in adults, where bones become soft due to inadequate mineralization. This condition can cause bone pain and muscle weakness, increasing the risk of fractures. In older adults, low vitamin D levels are strongly linked to an increased risk of osteoporosis and fractures.

Regular blood tests can help monitor your vitamin D levels, ensuring they remain within the optimal range. These tests measure the concentration of 25-hydroxyvitamin D in your blood, the best indicator of your vitamin D status. If your levels are low, your healthcare provider may recommend vitamin D supplements. These supplements come in two forms: vitamin D2 (ergocalciferol) and vitamin D3 (cholecalciferol). Vitamin D3 is generally more effective at raising blood levels of vitamin D and is the preferred form for supplementation.

Vitamin D is a cornerstone of bone health, working in tandem with calcium to maintain strong and resilient bones. By understanding the importance of this vitamin and ensuring you get enough through sunlight, diet, and supplements, you can significantly improve your bone density and reduce the risk of fractures.

3.3 PROTEIN AND BONE HEALTH: HOW MUCH DO YOU NEED?

Protein plays a vital role in maintaining bone health, particularly through its involvement in collagen formation. Collagen is the primary structural protein in bones, providing a scaffold that supports the deposition of minerals like calcium and phosphorus. This protein matrix is essential for giving bones their strength and flexibility. Without adequate protein, the formation and maintenance of this collagen network are compromised, leading to weaker bones and an increased risk of fractures. Moreover, protein contributes to muscle mass, which supports overall bone health. Strong muscles help stabilize joints and improve balance, reducing the likelihood of falls that could result in bone injuries.

For seniors, meeting daily protein requirements is crucial. The recommended dietary allowance (RDA) for protein is 0.8 grams per kilogram of body weight per day. However, as we age, our bodies become less efficient at utilizing protein, necessitating a higher intake. Many experts now recommend that older adults consume between 1.0 and 1.2 grams of protein per kilogram of body weight daily. For a person weighing 70 kilograms (154 pounds), this translates to 70 to 84 grams of protein each day. This increased intake ensures that your body has the necessary building blocks to maintain muscle mass and support bone health. If you have specific health conditions like kidney disease, consult your healthcare provider to determine the appropriate protein intake for your situation.

Incorporating high-protein foods into your diet can help you meet these increased needs. Lean meats such as chicken and turkey are excellent sources of high-quality protein. A 3-ounce serving of chicken breast provides about 26 grams of protein, making it a substantial contribution to your daily intake. Plant-based sources like beans, lentils, and tofu are also valuable. A cup of cooked lentils offers around 18 grams of protein, while half a cup of tofu provides roughly 10 grams. These options not only provide protein but also come with fiber and essential nutrients. Dairy products like Greek yogurt and cottage cheese are additional high-protein foods that can benefit bone health. A cup of Greek yogurt can contain up to 20 grams of protein, making it an excellent choice for a protein-packed snack or meal component.

Protein supplementation can be a practical solution if you struggle to meet your protein needs through diet alone. Various types of protein supplements are available, each with its own benefits. Whey protein is quickly absorbed and is ideal for post-exercise recovery, while casein provides a slower release of amino acids, making it suitable for sustained protein intake throughout the day. Plant-based protein supplements, such as those made from pea or soy protein, are excellent alternatives for those who prefer or need to avoid animal products. When considering protein supplements, follow guidelines for safe and effective use. Start with a modest amount and gradually increase it as needed, and always consult with your healthcare provider to ensure supplementation is appropriate for your dietary needs and health conditions.

Balancing protein intake throughout the day can enhance its benefits for both bone and muscle health. Instead of consuming most of your protein in one or two meals, aim to distribute it evenly across all meals and snacks. This approach ensures a steady supply of amino acids to support muscle protein synthesis and bone maintenance. For example, you might include eggs or Greek yogurt for breakfast, a turkey sandwich or lentil soup for lunch, and grilled chicken or tofu stir-fry for dinner. Adding protein-rich snacks like almonds, cheese, or protein shakes between meals can further help you meet your daily requirements.

Interactive Element: Protein Intake Checklist

To help you track and meet your daily protein intake, consider using this simple checklist:

- Breakfast: 2 eggs (12 grams) and a cup of Greek yogurt (20 grams)
- Lunch: Turkey sandwich (20 grams) and a cup of lentil soup (18 grams)
- Dinner: Grilled chicken breast (26 grams) with a side of quinoa (8 grams)
- Snacks: A handful of almonds (6 grams) and a protein shake (20 grams)

By following this checklist, you can ensure that you are consuming enough protein to support your bone health and overall well-being.

3.4 FOODS TO BOOST BONE HEALTH: A COMPREHENSIVE LIST

Maintaining strong bones requires more than just calcium and vitamin D. A well-rounded diet rich in various nutrients is crucial for optimal bone health. Incorporating a range of bone-healthy foods into your meals can significantly improve your bone density and overall well-being. Let's start with some of the most beneficial foods for bone health.

Dairy products like milk, cheese, and yogurt are well-known for their high calcium content, but they also provide other essential nutrients such as protein and phosphorus, which are vital for bone strength. Fortified plant milks, such as almond, soy, and rice milk, offer an excellent alternative for those who are lactose intolerant or prefer non-dairy options. These fortified beverages often contain added calcium and vitamin D, making them comparable to traditional dairy products in terms of bone health benefits.

Vitamin D is crucial for calcium absorption, and fatty fish like salmon is an excellent source. Salmon is not only rich in vitamin D but also provides omega-3 fatty acids, which have anti-inflammatory properties that can benefit overall bone health. Fortified cereals are another practical option for boosting your vitamin D intake. Many breakfast cereals are fortified with both calcium and vitamin D, making them an easy addition to your morning routine.

Magnesium is another essential nutrient for bone health as it plays a role in converting vitamin D into its active form, which aids calcium absorption. Foods rich in magnesium include nuts, seeds, and whole grains. Almonds, sunflower seeds, and flaxseeds are excellent choices that can be easily incorporated into your diet.

Whole grains like brown rice, quinoa, and whole wheat also provide magnesium and other nutrients that support bone health.

Some specific foods are particularly beneficial for bone health due to their high nutrient content. Sardines, for instance, are packed with both calcium and vitamin D. A serving of sardines can provide a significant portion of your daily calcium and vitamin D needs, making them a powerful ally in maintaining bone density. Sweet potatoes are another excellent choice, as they are rich in magnesium and potassium. Potassium helps neutralize acids that remove calcium from the body, thereby supporting bone health. Prunes, often overlooked, have been shown to help prevent bone loss. They are rich in antioxidants and nutrients like vitamin K and boron, which play roles in bone metabolism.

Incorporating these foods into your daily meals can be simple and enjoyable. Adding leafy greens like kale, spinach, or collard greens to smoothies is an easy way to boost your calcium intake without altering the flavor significantly. These greens can also be sautéed as a side dish or added to soups and stews. Using fortified plant milks in cooking and baking can seamlessly increase your intake of calcium and vitamin D. For example, substitute regular milk with almond or soy milk in recipes for pancakes, muffins, or creamy sauces.

Dietary diversity is crucial for ensuring all your nutrient needs are met. Rotating different protein sources throughout the week can help provide various essential amino acids and other nutrients. For instance, include lean meats, fish, beans, and tofu in your meal plans to ensure a balanced intake of protein and other bone-healthy nutrients. Trying new recipes that incorporate bone-healthy ingredients can keep your meals exciting and nutritious. Experiment with dishes like salmon and sweet potato bowls, quinoa and kale salads, or almond and prune energy bars.

Visual Element: Bone-Healthy Food Chart

Consider creating a chart that lists various bone-healthy foods along with their nutrient content. This visual aid can serve as a quick reference guide to help you plan balanced meals that support bone health. Here's an example:

- Dairy Products: Milk, cheese, yogurt (Calcium, Vitamin D, Protein)
- Fortified Plant Milks: Almond milk, soy milk (Calcium, Vitamin D)
- Fatty Fish: Salmon, mackerel (Vitamin D, Omega-3 Fatty Acids)
- Nuts and Seeds: Almonds, sunflower seeds, flaxseeds (Magnesium, Protein)
- Whole Grains: Brown rice, quinoa, whole wheat (Magnesium)
- Leafy Greens: Kale, spinach, collard greens (Calcium, Magnesium)
- Others: Sardines (Calcium, Vitamin D), Sweet Potatoes (Magnesium, Potassium), Prunes (Vitamin K, Antioxidants)

By incorporating various of these nutrient-rich foods into your diet, you can significantly enhance your bone health and overall well-being. This approach ensures that you receive all the essential nutrients needed to maintain strong and healthy bones.

3.5 MEAL PLANS FOR OPTIMAL BONE HEALTH

Creating meal plans tailored to support bone health can simplify your dietary choices and ensure you get the nutrients needed for strong bones. Let's start with breakfast, the meal that kickstarts your day. A bowl of calcium-fortified oatmeal paired with a side of fresh fruit provides a hearty start and delivers a good dose of bone-supporting calcium and fiber. The fortified oatmeal helps meet your calcium needs, while the fruit adds various vitamins and antioxidants. Consider adding a handful of nuts or seeds to your oatmeal for an extra boost of magnesium and healthy fats.

For lunch, a spinach and salmon salad with a light lemon dressing makes an excellent choice. Spinach is rich in calcium and other essential nutrients, while salmon provides a substantial amount of vitamin D and omega-3 fatty acids. These nutrients work together to enhance calcium absorption and reduce inflammation. The lemon dressing adds a refreshing flavor and contributes a bit of vitamin C, which aids in collagen formation, an important component of bone tissue. Adding some sliced almonds or sunflower seeds can enhance the nutrient profile and add a satisfying crunch.

Dinner could feature grilled chicken with quinoa and steamed broccoli. Chicken offers high-quality protein necessary for maintaining muscle mass and supporting bone health. Quinoa, a whole grain rich in magnesium, complements the chicken while providing additional protein and fiber. Steamed broccoli is an excellent source of calcium and vitamin K, another nutrient important for bone health. This balanced meal ensures you receive various nutrients that work synergistically to strengthen and maintain your bones.

Snacks play an equally important role in maintaining nutrient levels throughout the day. Greek yogurt with berries is a fantastic option. The yogurt provides protein and calcium, while the berries add antioxidants and vitamins. Another excellent snack choice is a handful of almonds paired with dried apricots. Almonds are rich in magnesium and healthy fats, while dried apricots offer fiber and a touch of natural sweetness. Cottage cheese with pineapple is another appealing option, combining protein-rich dairy with the vitamin C and fiber found in pineapple.

The timing of your meals can significantly impact nutrient absorption and overall health. Spreading nutrient intake throughout the day ensures that your body efficiently absorbs and utilizes the vitamins and minerals you consume. Balanced meals and snacks help maintain steady blood sugar levels, provide consistent energy, and support metabolic processes. Avoiding large, infrequent meals can prevent spikes and crashes in blood sugar levels, which can negatively affect your overall well-being. Consistent, smaller meals and snacks also help in better digestion and absorption of nutrients, ensuring that your body makes the most of what you eat.

To make meal planning easier, having a well-organized grocery list is essential. Here's a sample weekly grocery list for bone-healthy foods:

- Dairy: Milk, cheese, Greek yogurt, cottage cheese
- Vegetables: Spinach, kale, broccoli, sweet potatoes
- Protein: Chicken, salmon, lean turkey, tofu
- Whole grains: Quinoa, brown rice, fortified cereals
- Fruits: Berries, pineapple, dried apricots
- Nuts and seeds: Almonds, sunflower seeds, chia seeds
- Fortified foods: Orange juice, plant-based milks

Having these items on hand ensures you can prepare meals and snacks that support your bone health without much hassle. Let's look at some easy-to-follow recipes for each meal plan.

For breakfast, try making a bowl of calcium-fortified oatmeal. Combine half a cup of oatmeal with one cup of fortified milk and cook according to package instructions. Top with fresh berries and a tablespoon of chia seeds. For lunch, prepare a spinach and salmon salad. Start with a bed of fresh spinach, add a grilled salmon fillet, and top with sliced almonds and a light lemon dressing made from fresh lemon juice, olive oil, and a pinch of salt and pepper. For dinner, grill a chicken breast seasoned with your favorite herbs. Serve it alongside a cup of cooked quinoa and a serving of steamed broccoli, lightly seasoned with lemon juice and a dash of olive oil.

By incorporating these meal plans and snack ideas into your daily routine, you can ensure you are getting the necessary nutrients to support your bone health. The balanced intake of calcium, vitamin D, protein, magnesium, and other essential nutrients will help maintain strong bones and overall well-being. Planning your meals and snacks around these nutrient-rich foods makes it easier to meet your dietary needs and enjoy various delicious and healthy options.

4

SUPPLEMENT INFORMATION

When I first met Doris, she was a spirited 69-year-old who had always been diligent about her health. However, despite her active lifestyle and balanced diet, she was diagnosed with early-stage osteoporosis. Doris was puzzled and concerned. We discussed the potential gaps in her nutrition, and it became clear that she wasn't taking the right supplements to support her bone health. This conversation underscored the critical role that supplements can play in maintaining and improving bone density, especially as we age.

4.1 ESSENTIAL SUPPLEMENTS FOR BONE HEALTH: WHAT TO TAKE

To maintain strong bones and reduce the risk of fractures, certain supplements are particularly beneficial. Among the most critical are calcium, vitamin D, magnesium, and vitamin K2. Each of these supplements plays a unique and vital role in bone health, working together to ensure your bones remain resilient and strong.

Calcium is the cornerstone of bone health. It is essential for the formation and maintenance of bones. Your bones are the primary storage site for calcium in your body, and this mineral is crucial for maintaining bone density. Without adequate calcium, your body begins to withdraw this mineral from your bones, leading to weakened bone structure and increased fracture risk. For adults, the recommended daily intake of calcium is 1000 to 1200 milligrams, depending on age and gender. Women over 50 and men over 70 should aim for the higher end of this range to counteract the natural decline in bone density that comes with aging.

Vitamin D is another critical component for bone health. It aids in the absorption of calcium from the gut into the bloodstream. Without sufficient vitamin D, even a diet rich in calcium may not be enough to maintain strong bones. Vitamin D also plays a role in bone remodeling, ensuring that old bone is replaced by new bone tissue. The recommended daily intake of vitamin D is 800 to 1000 international units (IU) for adults. This dosage helps ensure that your body effectively absorbs the calcium you consume, supporting overall bone health.

Magnesium is often overlooked, but is equally important for maintaining bone density and strength. It plays a role in converting vitamin D into its active form, which aids calcium absorption. Magnesium also directly supports bone mineralization, contributing to the structural integrity of bones. For adults, the recommended daily intake of magnesium is 310 to 420 milligrams, depending on age and gender. Ensuring you get enough magnesium can help maintain bone density and support overall skeletal health.

Vitamin K2 is a lesser-known but crucial nutrient for bone health. It helps direct calcium to the bones where it is needed and away from the arteries, where it can cause harm. Vitamin K2 activates proteins that bind calcium, ensuring it is deposited in the bone matrix and not in the soft tissues or blood vessels. The recommended daily intake of vitamin K2 is 90 to 120 micrograms. This vitamin works synergistically with calcium and vitamin D to enhance bone density and reduce the risk of fractures.

When taking these supplements, it is essential to follow recommended dosages to avoid potential side effects. Calcium should be taken in doses of 1000 to 1200 milligrams per day. Exceeding this amount can lead to kidney stones and interfere with the absorption of other essential minerals. Vitamin D should be consumed in doses of 800 to 1000 IU daily. Too much vitamin D can cause toxicity, leading to symptoms like nausea, weakness, and kidney damage. Magnesium should be taken in doses of 310 to 420 milligrams per day. High doses of magnesium can cause digestive issues such as diarrhea and abdominal cramping. Vitamin K2 should be taken in doses of 90 to 120 micrograms per day. While vitamin K2 toxicity is rare, it is still essential to adhere to recommended dosages.

Safety is paramount when taking supplements. Avoid megadoses unless prescribed by a healthcare provider, as excessive intake can lead to adverse effects and interactions with medications. Always check for potential interactions with your current medications. For example, calcium can interfere with the absorption of certain antibiotics and thyroid medications. Consult your healthcare provider before starting any new supplement to ensure it is safe and beneficial for your specific health needs. They can provide personalized recommendations based on your medical history and current health status.

Interactive Element: Supplement Tracking Chart

To help you manage your supplement intake effectively, consider using a supplement tracking chart. This simple tool allows you to record the type, dosage, and timing of each supplement you take. Here's a sample layout:

- Calcium: 1000-1200 mg per day
    - Type: _____
    - Dosage: _____
    - Timing: _____
- Vitamin D: 800-1000 IU per day
    - Type: _____
    - Dosage: _____
    - Timing: _____
- Magnesium: 310-420 mg per day
    - Type: _____
    - Dosage: _____
    - Timing: _____
- Vitamin K2: 90-120 mcg per day
    - Type: _____
    - Dosage: _____
    - Timing: _____

By keeping track of your supplement intake, you can ensure you are meeting your daily requirements and monitor for any potential interactions or side effects. This proactive approach helps maintain optimal bone health and overall well-being.

4.2 CALCIUM SUPPLEMENTS: DOSAGES AND BEST PRACTICES

Calcium supplements come in various forms, each with its own advantages and considerations. The most common types include calcium carbonate, calcium citrate, and less frequently, calcium lactate and calcium gluconate. Each form has unique properties that may make it more suitable for your specific needs. Calcium carbonate, for instance, contains the highest percentage of elemental calcium, about 40%. This makes it a potent option, but it is best absorbed when taken with food. Calcium carbonate may cause mild gastrointestinal discomfort, such as constipation or bloating, but for many, the cost-effectiveness and availability make it a popular choice.

Calcium citrate, on the other hand, contains about 21% elemental calcium. Although it has a lower calcium content per pill, it is more easily absorbed by the body, even on an empty stomach. This makes calcium citrate a suitable option for those taking acid-reducing medications or who have digestive issues. It tends to be gentler on the stomach, reducing the likelihood of gastrointestinal side effects. Calcium lactate and calcium gluconate are less common but still valuable options. They contain lower percentages of elemental calcium, around 13% and 9%, respectively. These forms are often used in liquid supplements or for those who require very gentle supplementation due to severe digestive issues.

When choosing the right calcium supplement, several factors should guide your decision. Absorption rates vary significantly between the different forms of calcium. If you have a history of digestive discomfort or are taking medications that affect stomach acidity, calcium citrate might be the best option for you due to its superior absorption rate in such conditions. Tolerance and digestive comfort are also crucial considerations. If you've experienced constipation or bloating with calcium carbonate, switching to calcium citrate or a liquid form of calcium lactate or gluconate may alleviate these issues. Cost and availability are practical concerns as well. Calcium carbonate is generally the most affordable and widely available, making it a convenient choice for many. However, the slightly higher cost of calcium citrate might be worth it for the increased comfort and absorption benefits.

Proper dosing of calcium supplements is essential to maximize their benefits and minimize side effects. It is generally recommended to divide your calcium intake throughout the day, as your body absorbs calcium most efficiently in smaller amounts. Aim to take no more than 500 milligrams of calcium at a time. This approach ensures that your body can fully absorb the calcium and reduces the risk of side effects like constipation. If you're taking calcium carbonate, it's best to take it with meals to enhance absorption. In contrast, calcium citrate can be taken with or without food, providing more flexibility. The recommended daily intake of calcium varies by age and gender. For adults, a daily intake of 1000 to 1200 milligrams is advised, with women over 50 and men over 70 aiming for the higher end of this range.

While calcium supplements are generally safe, they can cause side effects if not taken correctly. Constipation is a common issue, particularly with calcium carbonate. Increasing your water and fiber intake can help mitigate this problem. Foods rich in fiber, such as fruits, vegetables, and whole grains, can ease digestive discomfort and promote regularity. Staying well-hydrated also supports digestive health and helps prevent constipation. Kidney stones are another potential side effect of excessive calcium supplementation. Ensuring adequate hydration is crucial to minimize this risk. Drinking plenty of water helps flush excess calcium from your kidneys, reducing the likelihood of stone formation.

Calcium supplements can also interfere with the absorption of other essential minerals, such as iron and zinc. To minimize this interaction, it's advisable to take calcium supplements at a different time than other mineral supplements or medications. For instance, if you take an iron supplement or a thyroid medication, try to space it at least two hours apart from your calcium supplement. This spacing allows your body to absorb each nutrient more effectively, ensuring you get the full benefit of each supplement.

Interactive Element: Calcium Supplement Checklist

To help you choose and manage your calcium supplement intake effectively, consider using this checklist:

- Calcium Carbonate:
    - Advantages: High elemental calcium, cost-effective
    - Best taken with food
    - Potential side effects: Constipation, bloating
- Calcium Citrate:
    - Advantages: Easier absorption, suitable for those with digestive issues
    - It can be taken with or without food
    - Gentle on the stomach
- Calcium Lactate/Gluconate:
    - Advantages: Suitable for liquid supplements
    - Lower elemental calcium, gentle on the stomach
    - Ideal for those with severe digestive issues
- Dosing Tips:
    - Divide doses throughout the day (no more than 500 mg at a time)
    - Increase water and fiber intake to prevent constipation
    - Ensure adequate hydration to prevent kidney stones

- Take at different times from other mineral supplements or medications

By following these guidelines and using this checklist, you can ensure you are selecting the most suitable calcium supplement for your needs and taking it in a way that maximizes its benefits while minimizing any potential side effects. This proactive approach will help you maintain strong and healthy bones, supporting your overall well-being.

4.3 VITAMIN D SUPPLEMENTS: CHOOSING THE RIGHT ONE

Vitamin D is a critical nutrient for bone health, but not all forms of vitamin D are created equal. There are two primary forms of vitamin D supplements: vitamin D2 (ergocalciferol) and vitamin D3 (cholecalciferol). Vitamin D2 is plant-based, commonly derived from sources like mushrooms and yeast. It is often used in fortified foods and some over-the-counter supplements. Vitamin D3, on the other hand, is animal-based, typically sourced from lanolin in sheep's wool or fish oil. Research indicates that vitamin D3 is more effective at raising and maintaining vitamin D levels in the blood compared to vitamin D2. This increased effectiveness makes vitamin D3 the preferred choice for most individuals looking to improve their vitamin D status and, consequently, their bone health.

Finding the right vitamin D supplement can be straightforward, given the variety of options available. Over-the-counter vitamin D supplements are widely accessible and come in various forms, including tablets, capsules, and liquid drops. These options are convenient and can be easily incorporated into your daily routine. For those with severe vitamin D deficiency or specific medical conditions, prescription-strength vitamin D supplements may be necessary. These higher-dose supplements are typically prescribed by healthcare providers and are used to correct significant deficiencies more rapidly. In addition to supplements, fortified foods can also help boost your vitamin D intake. Many dairy products, plant-based milks, and cereals are fortified with vitamin D, providing an additional source of this vital nutrient in your diet.

Dosing guidelines for vitamin D supplements can vary based on individual needs and current vitamin D levels. For maintaining adequate levels, a standard daily dosage of 800 to 1000 international units (IU) is generally recommended for adults. However, if you have a diagnosed deficiency, higher doses may be necessary to bring your levels up to a healthy range. In such cases, healthcare providers might recommend doses ranging from 2000 to 4000 IU per day or even higher in some instances. The frequency of dosing can also vary; while daily supplementation is common, some individuals may benefit from weekly or even monthly high-dose vitamin D supplements, depending on their specific needs and medical advice.

Maximizing the absorption of vitamin D supplements is crucial for ensuring you get the full benefit. Vitamin D is a fat-soluble vitamin, meaning it is best absorbed when taken with meals containing fat. Including healthy fats in your diet, such as those found in avocados, nuts, and olive oil, can enhance absorption. Consistent sunlight exposure is another important factor. Spending time outdoors in natural sunlight helps your body produce vitamin D naturally. Even short periods of sun exposure can make a difference, especially during the sunnier months. Monitoring your blood levels of vitamin D through regular check-ups can help you and your healthcare provider adjust your dosage as needed, ensuring you maintain optimal levels for bone health.

Interactive Element: Vitamin D Supplement Checklist

To help you choose the right vitamin D supplement and ensure you are maximizing its benefits, consider using this checklist:

- Vitamin D2 (ergocalciferol):
  - Plant-based
  - Common in fortified foods and some supplements
  - Less effective at raising blood levels
- Vitamin D3 (cholecalciferol):
  - Animal-based, more effective
  - Sourced from lanolin or fish oil
  - Preferred choice for supplementation
- Sources of Vitamin D Supplements:
  - Over-the-counter options: Tablets, capsules, liquid drops
  - Prescription-strength supplements: Higher doses for deficiency correction
  - Fortified foods: Dairy products, plant-based milks, cereals
- Dosing Guidelines:
  - Standard maintenance dose: 800-1000 IU per day
  - Deficiency correction: 2000-4000 IU per day, or as prescribed
  - Frequency: Daily, weekly, or monthly, based on medical advice
- Absorption Tips:
  - Take with meals containing fat
  - Ensure consistent sunlight exposure
  - Monitor blood levels regularly to adjust dosage

By following these guidelines and using this checklist, you can effectively manage your vitamin D intake, ensuring you receive the full benefits for your bone health.

4.4 UNDERSTANDING MULTIVITAMINS AND THEIR IMPACT ON BONE HEALTH

Multivitamins are dietary supplements that combine various essential vitamins and minerals into one convenient form. They are designed to fill dietary gaps, ensuring that you receive the necessary nutrients that might be missing from your diet. As we age, it becomes increasingly important to maintain a balanced intake of these nutrients to support overall health, including bone health. Multivitamins typically come in various forms, such as pills, capsules, powders, and liquids, each offering a mix of vitamins like A, C, D, E, and minerals such as calcium, magnesium, and zinc.

The effectiveness of multivitamins in supporting bone health lies in their convenience and ability to provide a broad spectrum of nutrients in one supplement. This can simplify your daily routine, especially if you find it challenging to consume a varied diet rich in all the necessary vitamins and minerals. However, multivitamins may not always contain adequate dosages of specific nutrients needed for optimal bone health. For example, while a multivitamin might include calcium and vitamin D, the amounts may be insufficient to meet the recommended daily intake for seniors. This limitation means that relying solely on multivitamins may not fully address your bone health needs.

Choosing a high-quality multivitamin requires careful consideration. Look for a product with a comprehensive ingredient list that includes essential vitamins and minerals tailored to your age and health needs. Avoid multivitamins with unnecessary additives, such as artificial colors, flavors, or fillers, as these do not contribute to your health and may even cause adverse reactions. The dosages of each nutrient should be appropriate for seniors, considering the increased needs for certain vitamins and minerals. For instance, ensure that the multivitamin provides adequate levels of vitamin D and calcium, which are crucial for maintaining bone density.

Another critical aspect of taking multivitamins is understanding their potential interactions with other medications and supplements. Nutrient overlap can occur, leading to excessive intake of certain vitamins or minerals, which can be harmful. For example, if you are already taking a separate calcium supplement, ensure that your multivitamin does not push your total calcium intake beyond the safe limit. Consulting with your healthcare provider is essential before starting any new supplement regimen. They can help you navigate potential interactions and recommend a multivitamin that complements your existing medications and supplements.

Safety is paramount when incorporating multivitamins into your routine. Avoid megadoses, as high levels of certain nutrients can cause toxicity and adverse health effects. For instance, excessive vitamin A can lead to liver damage and bone loss, while too much iron can cause gastrointestinal issues and interfere with the absorption of other minerals. Stick to the recommended dosages and regularly review your supplement intake with your healthcare provider to ensure it remains appropriate for your changing health needs.

Understanding the role and proper use of multivitamins can significantly enhance your bone health strategy. While they offer a convenient way to ensure you receive a broad spectrum of nutrients, it is vital to choose a high-quality product and be mindful of potential interactions with other medications and supplements. Consulting with your healthcare provider will help you make informed decisions, ensuring that your supplement regimen supports your overall health and bone density.

In the next chapter, we will delve into practical tips and strategies for daily bone health management. This will include setting realistic goals, tracking progress, and staying motivated.

5

DETAILED EXERCISE ROUTINES

Years ago, I worked with a gentleman named Harold, who had always been an active gardener. However, as he aged, he noticed that he couldn't lift heavy bags of soil or spend as much time tending his plants without feeling pain in his joints. When we started incorporating bone-building exercises into his routine, he experienced a remarkable improvement in his strength and stamina. This transformation reinforced the power of targeted exercise in maintaining and improving bone health, especially for seniors.

5.1 BONE-BUILDING WORKOUTS: INTRODUCTION AND BENEFITS

Bone-building exercises are activities specifically designed to strengthen your bones and improve overall skeletal health. These exercises fall into two main categories: weight-bearing exercises and resistance training. Weight-bearing exercises involve activities where you move against gravity while staying upright. Examples include walking, jogging, dancing, and climbing stairs. These activities put stress on your bones, prompting them to increase their density and strength. Resistance training, on the other hand, involves activities that use resistance to strengthen your muscles and bones. This can be achieved through weight lifting, using resistance bands, or performing body-weight exercises like push-ups and squats.

Incorporating bone-building workouts into your daily routine provides numerous benefits. One of the most significant advantages is increased bone density. As you engage in weight-bearing and resistance exercises, your bones respond to the stress by becoming denser, which reduces the risk of fractures. Improved muscle strength is another critical benefit. Strong muscles support your joints and bones, making daily activities easier and reducing the likelihood of falls. Enhanced balance and coordination are additional advantages. These exercises improve your overall stability, which is crucial for preventing falls and maintaining independence as you age.

Safety is paramount when performing bone-building exercises. To ensure you exercise safely, always start with proper warm-up routines. A warm-up prepares your muscles and joints for physical activity, reducing the risk of injury. Simple activities like brisk walking or gentle stretching for 5-10 minutes can effectively warm up your body. Similarly, cooling down after exercise is essential. This helps your body transition back to a resting state and reduces muscle soreness. Gentle stretching or a slow walk for 5-10 minutes can serve as an effective cool-down routine.

Using correct form and technique during exercises is crucial for maximizing benefits and preventing injuries. Pay attention to your body's alignment and movements. If you're unsure about the correct form, consider working with a fitness trainer or using instructional videos. Listening to your body is equally important.

Exercise should challenge you but not cause pain. If you feel sharp pain or discomfort, stop immediately and consult a healthcare professional. Overexertion can lead to injuries, so it's essential to balance effort with safety.

There are several misconceptions about bone-building exercises that often deter seniors from participating. One common myth is that weight-bearing exercises are too intense for older adults. In reality, there are modified versions of these exercises suitable for all fitness levels. For instance, if jogging is too strenuous, brisk walking or dancing can be effective alternatives. Resistance training is often misunderstood as requiring heavy weights, but resistance bands or light hand weights can provide sufficient resistance to strengthen muscles and bones without causing strain.

ature Visual Element: Exercise Safety Checklist

- Warm-Up Routine:
  - Brisk walking or gentle stretching for 5-10 minutes.
- Cool-Down Routine:
  - Gentle stretching or slow walk for 5-10 minutes.
- Correct Form and Technique:
  - Pay attention to body alignment.
  - Consider working with a fitness trainer or using instructional videos.
- Listening to Your Body:
  - Exercise should challenge but not cause pain.
  - Stop immediately if you feel sharp pain or discomfort.
  - Consult a healthcare professional if necessary.

By following these guidelines and incorporating bone-building exercises into your routine, you can significantly improve your bone health, muscle strength, and overall well-being.

5.2 BEGINNER EXERCISE ROUTINES: STEP-BY-STEP GUIDE

When starting a new exercise routine, it's important to begin with a structured plan that suits your current fitness level. A beginner exercise routine should include a balanced combination of warm-up exercises, core strengthening activities, and cool-down stretches to ensure a comprehensive approach to enhancing bone health and overall fitness.

Start your routine with warm-up exercises to prepare your body for more strenuous activities. Warm-ups increase blood flow to your muscles, making them more flexible and reducing the risk of injury. Begin with marching in place for about 10 minutes. This simple activity gets your heart rate up and warms up your leg muscles. Stand tall with your feet hip-width apart. Lift your knees to waist level, one at a time, as if you were marching. Swing your arms naturally to maintain balance. If you feel wobbly, do this near a wall or sturdy chair for support.

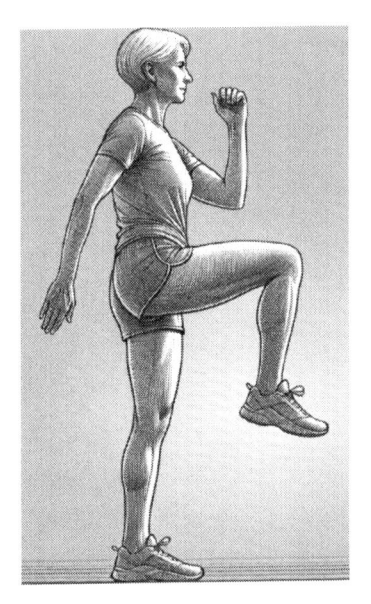

Fig 5.1 Marching in place

Once you are warmed up, move on to core exercises that focus on building strength and stability. Chair squats are an excellent starting point. Stand in front of a sturdy chair with your feet shoulder-width apart. Slowly bend your knees and lower your hips as if you were going to sit down. Keep your back straight and your weight on your heels. Lightly touch the chair with your bottom, then stand back up. Perform 2 sets of 10 repetitions. This exercise strengthens your quadriceps, hamstrings, and glutes, which are crucial for maintaining mobility and balance.

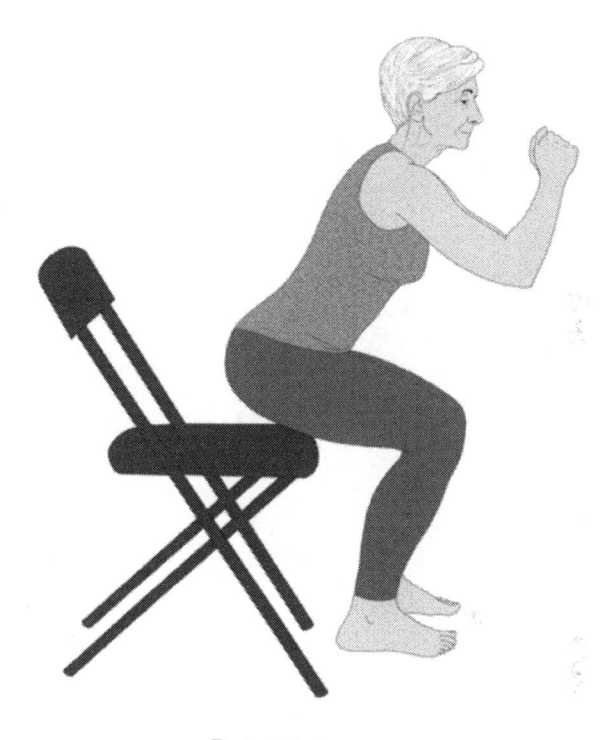

Fig 5.2 Chair squats

Another effective core exercise is the table push-up. Stand about an arm's length away from a counter or table. Place your hands on the table at shoulder height and shoulder-width apart. Keep your body straight from head to heels. Bend your elbows to bring your chest towards the table, then push back to the starting position. Perform 2 sets of 10 repetitions. Table push-ups work your chest, shoulders, and triceps, and are a safer alternative to traditional push-ups for those just starting out.

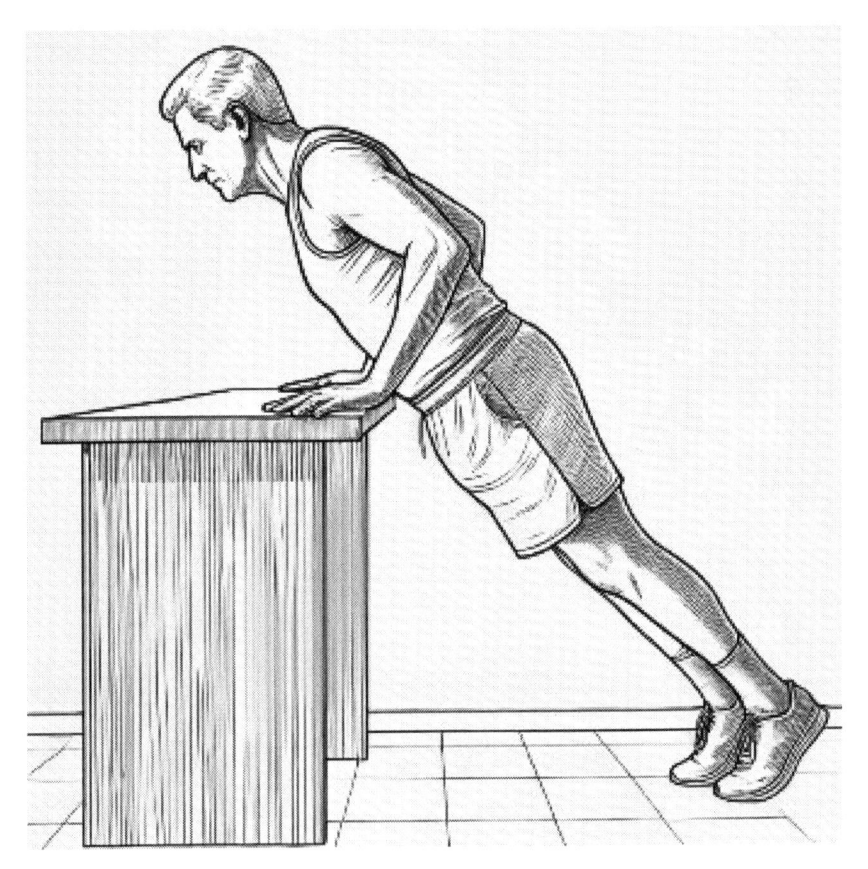

Fig 5.3 Table push-up

After completing the core exercises, it's important to cool down with stretches to help your muscles recover and maintain flexibility. Gentle stretching can reduce muscle soreness and improve your range of motion. Start with a standing quad stretch. Hold on to a wall or chair for balance. Bend one knee to bring your heel towards your buttocks and grasp your ankle with your hand. Hold the stretch for 20-30 seconds, then switch legs. Repeat for both sides. Follow this with a seated hamstring stretch. Sit on the edge of a chair with one leg extended straight out and the other foot flat on another chair. Reach towards the toes of the extended leg while keeping your back straight. Hold for 20-30 seconds, then switch legs.

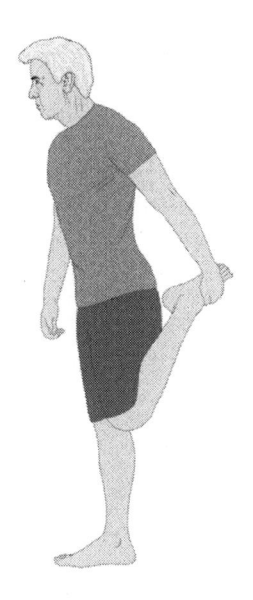

Fig 5.4 Standing quad stretch

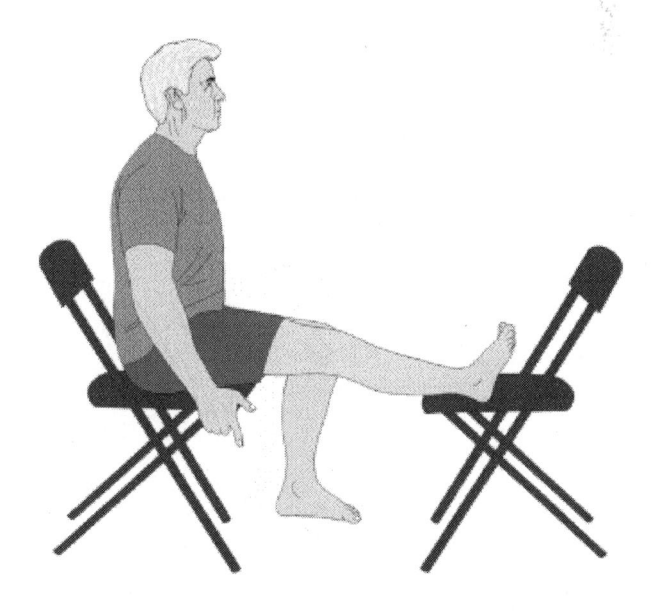

Fig 5.5 Seated hamstring stretch

For those with limited mobility, modifications can make these exercises more accessible. Seated leg lifts are a great alternative to marching in place. Sit tall in a sturdy chair with your feet flat on the floor. Lift one leg straight out in front of you, hold for a few seconds, then lower it back down. Alternate legs and perform 2 sets of 10 repetitions. This exercise strengthens your quadriceps without putting strain on your joints. Similarly, arm circles while sitting can serve as a modification for wall push-ups. Sit with your arms lifted out to the sides at shoulder height. Make small circles with your arms, gradually making them larger. Perform this for 1-2 minutes. This activity works your shoulder muscles and improves flexibility.

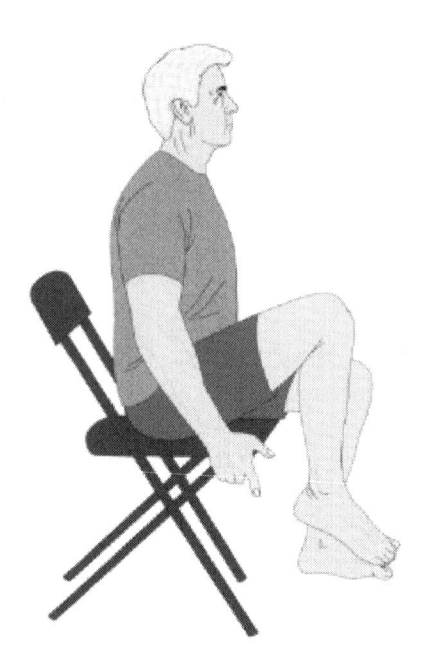

Fig 5.6 Seated leg lifts

DETAILED EXERCISE ROUTINES | 75

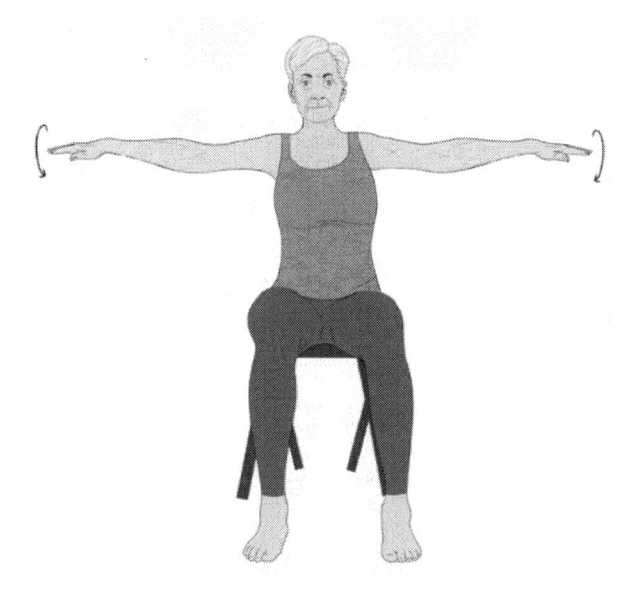

Fig 5.7 Seated arm circles

Interactive Element: Beginner Exercise Routine Checklist

- Warm-Up:
    - Marching in place for 10 minutes.
- Core Exercises:
    - Chair squats: 2 sets of 10 repetitions.
    - Table push-ups: 2 sets of 10 repetitions.
- Cool-Down Stretches:
    - Standing quad stretch: Hold for 20-30 seconds on each leg.
    - Seated hamstring stretch: Hold for 20-30 seconds on each leg.
- Modifications for Limited Mobility:
    - Seated leg lifts: 2 sets of 10 repetitions.
    - Arm circles while seated: Perform for 1-2 minutes.

76 | COMPREHENSIVE BONE HEALTH STRATEGIES

By following this beginner exercise routine, you can build a strong foundation for improving your bone health and overall fitness.

5.3 INTERMEDIATE EXERCISE ROUTINES: STEP-BY-STEP GUIDE

As you progress in your fitness journey, it's time to incorporate more challenging exercises into your routine. An intermediate-level exercise routine builds on the foundation you've established with beginner exercises, adding more dynamic movements and resistance to further enhance your strength and bone health. This routine should start with dynamic warm-up exercises, followed by core and balance exercises, and conclude with cool-down stretches.

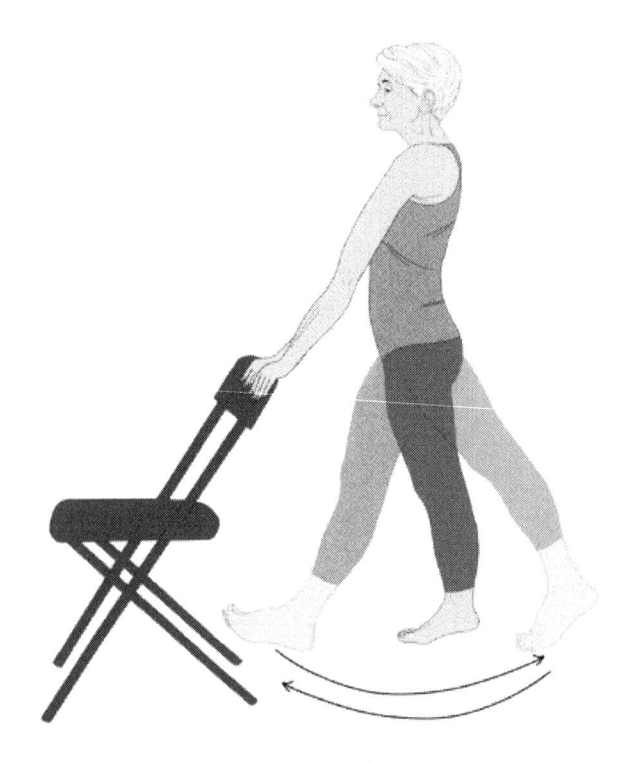

Fig 5.8 Leg swings

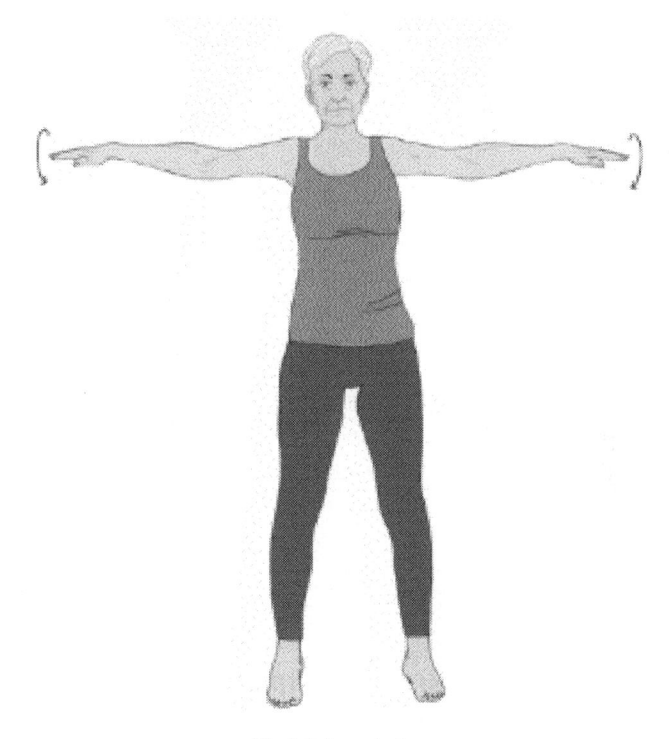

Fig 5.9 Arm circles

Begin your routine with dynamic warm-up exercises to prepare your muscles and joints for more intense activity. Dynamic warm-ups involve active movements that increase your heart rate and improve your range of motion. Start with leg swings. Stand next to a wall or chair for support. Swing one leg forward and backward, gradually increasing the range of motion. Perform 10 swings per leg. Follow this with arm circles. Extend your arms out to the sides at shoulder height and make small circles, gradually making them larger. Perform this for 1-2 minutes. Lastly, incorporate some hip circles. Stand with your feet hip-width apart and place your hands on your hips. Make circular motions with your hips, first clockwise, then counterclockwise. Do 10 circles in each direction.

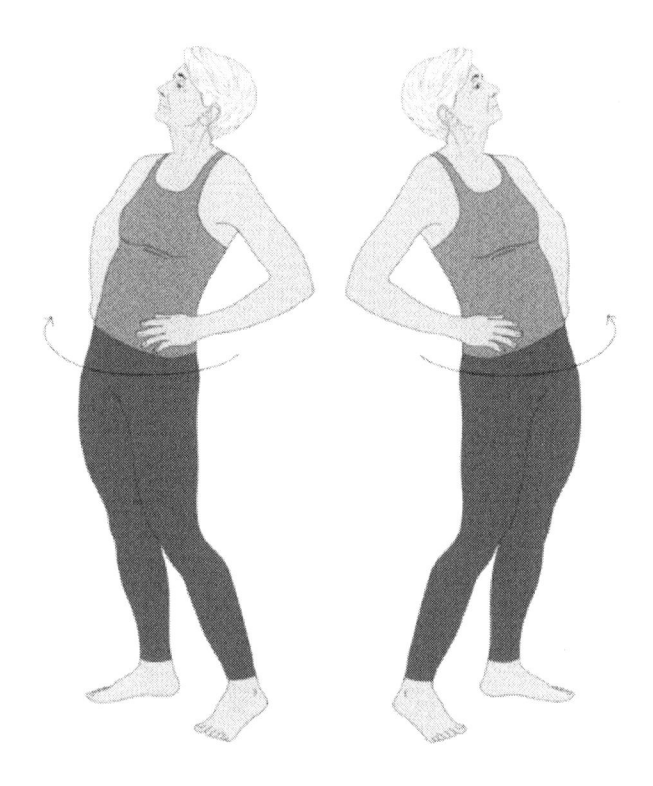

Fig 5.10 Hip circles

After warming up, move on to core and balance exercises that challenge your strength and stability. Step-ups are an excellent exercise for this purpose. Find a sturdy bench or step about knee height. Step onto the bench with your right foot, then bring your left foot up to meet it. Step back down with your right foot, followed by your left. Perform 2 sets of 10 repetitions per leg. This exercise targets your quadriceps, hamstrings, and glutes, enhancing your lower body strength and balance.

DETAILED EXERCISE ROUTINES | 79

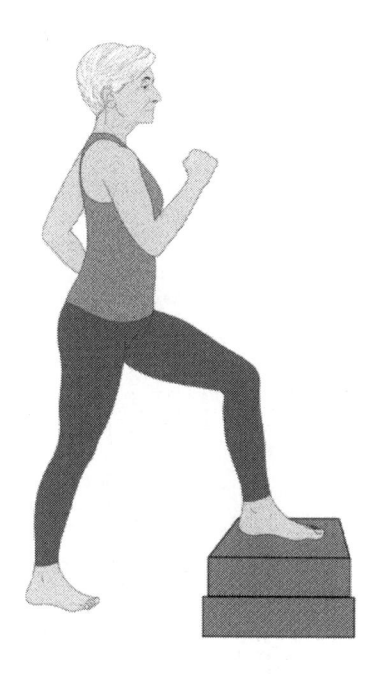

Fig 5.11 Step-ups

Next, incorporate resistance band bicep curls to build upper body strength. Stand in the middle of a resistance band with your feet shoulder-width apart. Hold the handles or ends of the band with your palms facing forward. Keeping your elbows close to your body, curl your hands up towards your shoulders, then slowly lower them back down. Perform 2 sets of 12 repetitions. This exercise strengthens your biceps and forearms, which are crucial for everyday tasks like lifting and carrying objects.

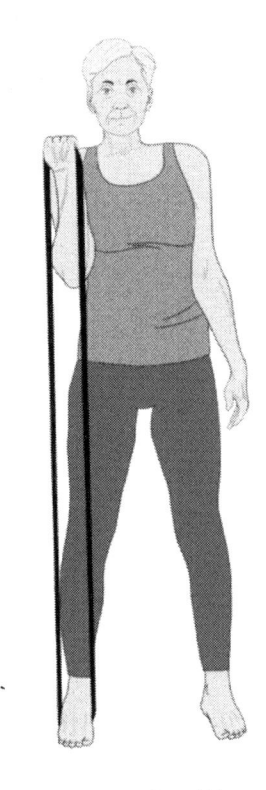

Fig 5.12 Resistance band bicep curls

Standing calf raises are another effective exercise for building lower leg strength. Stand holding a sturdy chair with your feet flat on the floor. Lift your heels off the ground as high as possible, then slowly lower them back down. Perform 2 sets of 12 repetitions. This exercise targets your calf muscles, improving your overall lower body strength and stability.

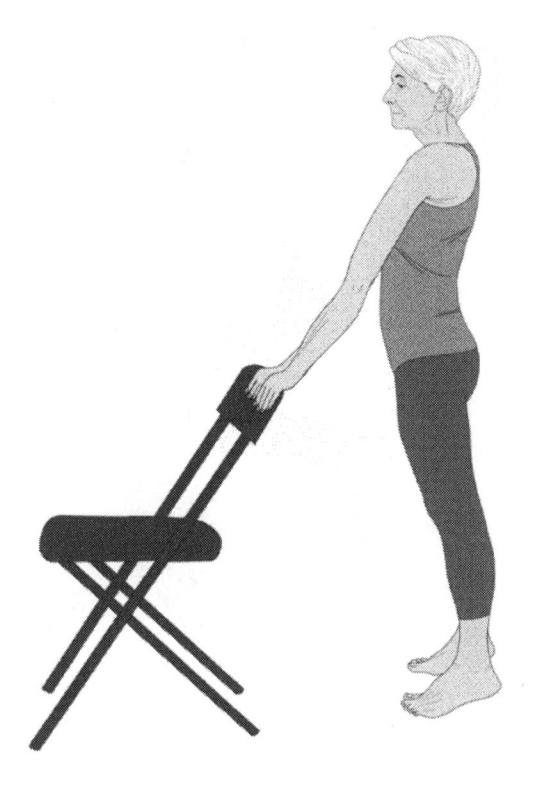

Fig 5.13 Standing calf raises

Transitioning from beginner to intermediate exercises involves gradually increasing the intensity of your workouts. Start by adding more repetitions or sets to your existing exercises. For example, if you've been doing 2 sets of 10 repetitions, try increasing to 3 sets of 12 repetitions. Incorporating resistance bands or light weights can also add a new level of challenge. Resistance bands are versatile and can be used for various exercises, providing adjustable resistance that can be tailored to your fitness level. Light weights, such as dumbbells, can be gradually increased as you build strength.

To ensure a smooth transition, listen to your body and make adjustments as needed. If an exercise feels too challenging, reduce the resistance or number of repetitions. Conversely, if an exercise feels too easy, increase the resistance or add more repetitions. It's essential to find a balance that challenges you without causing strain or injury.

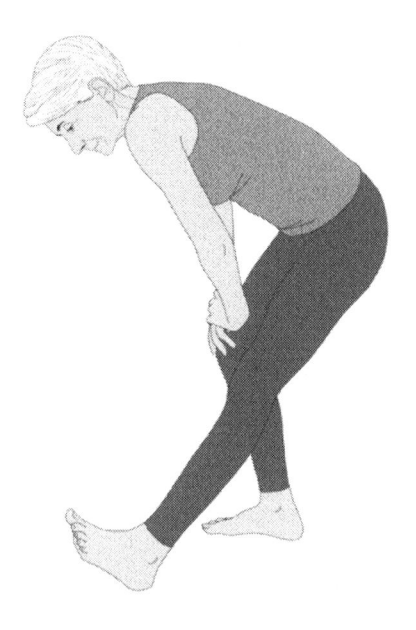

Fig 5.14 Standing hamstring stretch

Cool-down stretches are crucial for helping your muscles recover and maintaining flexibility. After completing your core and balance exercises, spend a few minutes on gentle stretching. Begin with a standing hamstring stretch. Stand with your feet hip-width apart and bend at the hips to reach towards your toes. Hold for 20-30 seconds. Follow this with a seated spinal twist. Sit on the edge of a chair with your feet flat on the floor. Place your right hand on the back of the chair and twist your torso to the right, looking over your shoulder. Hold for 20-30 seconds, then switch sides.

Finish with a calf stretch. Stand facing a wall with your hands against it at shoulder height. Step one foot back and press your heel into the ground, feeling a stretch in your calf. Hold for 20-30 seconds, then switch legs.

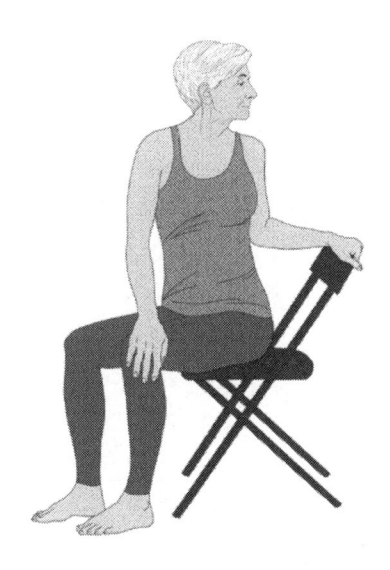

Fig 5.14 Seated spinal twist

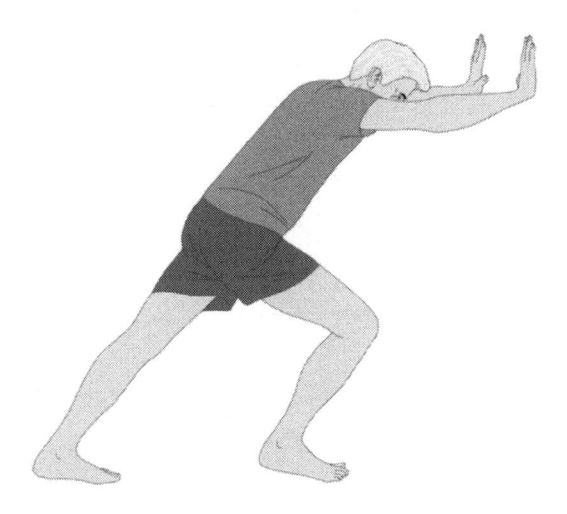

Fig 5.15 Calf stretch

84 | COMPREHENSIVE BONE HEALTH STRATEGIES

By following this intermediate exercise routine, you can continue to build on your progress, enhancing your strength, balance, and overall bone health.

5.4 ADVANCED EXERCISE ROUTINES: STEP-BY-STEP GUIDE

For those ready to take their fitness to the next level, an advanced exercise routine offers more challenging activities to build strength, enhance flexibility, and improve overall bone health. This routine should begin with comprehensive warm-up exercises to prepare your body for high-intensity movements. Start with dynamic stretches such as leg swings and arm circles, which can increase your range of motion and reduce the risk of injury. Adding movements like jumping jacks or high knees can further elevate your heart rate and ensure your muscles are adequately warmed up.

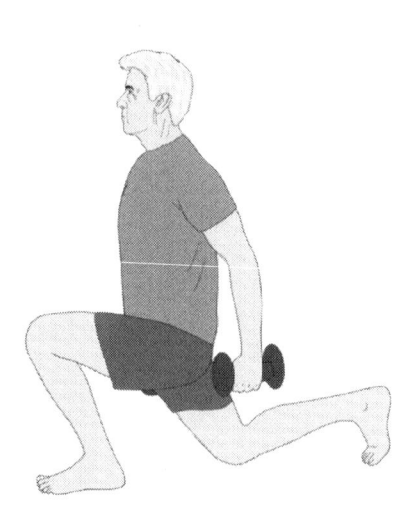

Fig 5.16 Weighted lunges

DETAILED EXERCISE ROUTINES | 85

Once you are warmed up, transition to high-intensity core and strength exercises. Weighted lunges are an excellent starting point. To perform a weighted lunge, stand upright with a dumbbell in each hand, arms at your sides. Step forward with your right leg and lower your body until your right thigh is parallel to the ground, keeping your knee directly above your ankle. Push back to the starting position and repeat. Perform 3 sets of 12 repetitions per leg. This exercise targets the quadriceps, hamstrings, and glutes, providing a comprehensive lower body workout.

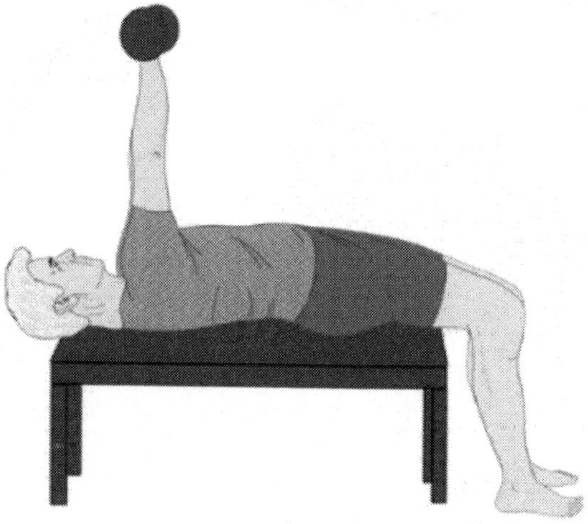

Fig 5.17 Dumbbell chest press

Next, incorporate the dumbbell chest press to strengthen your upper body. Lie on your back on a flat bench with a dumbbell in each hand. Position the dumbbells at chest level, palms facing forward. Press the weights upward until your arms are fully extended, then lower them back to the starting position. Ensure controlled movements throughout the exercise to maximize muscle activation and reduce the risk of injury. Perform 3 sets of 10 repetitions. This exercise primarily targets the pectoral muscles, triceps, and shoulders, contributing to overall upper body strength.

Plank holds are another crucial component of an advanced routine. Position yourself in a forearm plank position, with elbows directly under your shoulders and your body forming a straight line from head to heels. Engage your core muscles and hold this position for 30 seconds. Gradually increase the duration as your strength improves. Perform 3 sets of 30 seconds. Planks are excellent for building core stability and strength, which is vital for maintaining good posture and balance.

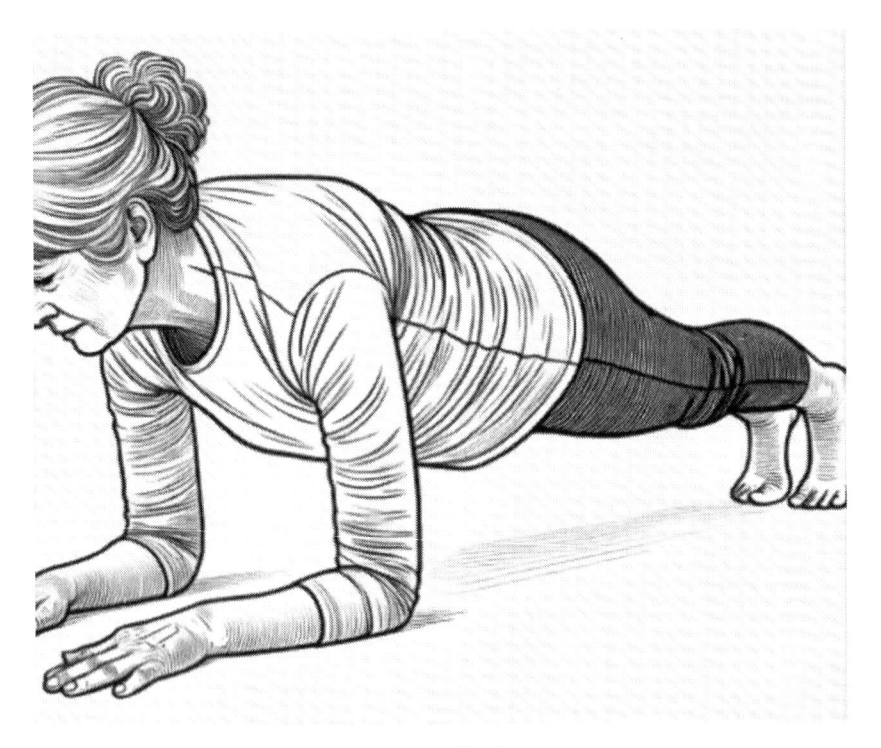

Fig 5.18 Plank

Maintaining proper form is crucial to prevent injuries and ensure you get the most out of your exercises. Using mirrors or seeking feedback from a workout partner can help you maintain correct form. Controlled movements are essential; avoid rushing through exercises, as this can lead to improper technique and increase the risk of injury. Focus on slow, deliberate movements to engage the targeted muscles effectively. Additionally, pay attention to your body's signals. If you experience pain or discomfort, stop immediately and consult a healthcare professional.

Visual aids can be incredibly helpful in mastering advanced exercises. Consider linking to demonstration videos to ensure you understand the correct form and technique. These visual aids can serve as valuable resources, helping you perform exercises safely and effectively.

Weighted lunges require precision to avoid strain on the knees. Keep your back straight and your core engaged throughout the movement. Dumbbell chest presses demand a secure grip and controlled breathing. Exhale as you press the weights up, and inhale as you lower them. Plank holds necessitate a strong core and flat back; avoid letting your hips sag or pike upward. By focusing on these details, you can perform advanced exercises with confidence and minimize the risk of injury.

An advanced exercise routine can significantly enhance your strength, flexibility, and overall bone health. Starting with comprehensive warm-ups, progressing through high-intensity core and strength exercises, and ending with cool-down stretches ensures a balanced and effective workout. Paying attention to proper form and using visual aids can further enhance your exercise experience, helping you achieve your fitness goals safely and efficiently.

Stop Osteoporosis From Silently Creeping Up on Others

"The tradition has been to think that aging causes bone weakness... It turns out that the reverse is also largely true: loss of bone density and degradation of the health of the bones also causes aging, diabetes, and, for males, loss of fertility and sexual function. We just cannot isolate any causal relationship in a complex system."

— NASSIM NICHOLAS TALEB

Before you continue your reading journey, I'd love to tell you a story that demonstrates how quietly bone issues can creep up on you. Actress Brit Eckland recalls having been diagnosed with osteoporosis quite by chance when she was aged 53. She felt horrified, as she was a healthy, fit, and energetic mom of an eight-year-old daughter.

Her reaction is not uncommon. Many patients share the same sense of shock when they discover that their bone density is not what it should be for their age. From the start of this book, I have aimed to shed light on why osteoporosis can be a silent enemy that often shows no symptoms at all until much later in life. The good news is that osteoporosis (or osteopenia) can be treated and effectively prevented.

Thus far, I have shown how easy and painless it is to obtain a bone scan, which reveals the state of your bone health in a matter of minutes. I have also discussed the main prescription medications for osteoporosis and arthritis and revealed the major difference that a bone-focused diet and bone-building workout can have. If you have already started making these changes in your life, I bet you can't wait to get to the next chapter, which is all about how to be consistent, stay motivated, and prevent falls. If so, please do me one small favor—let others know what you think of this book so far!

By leaving a review of this book on Amazon, you'll let new readers know that testing and prevention are important—even if they are in their 30s or even younger.

Thanks for your help. Osteoporosis and osteopenia don't have to be silent enemies if we identify them and stop them in their tracks before they even get close to wreaking havoc.

Scan the QR code below

6

PRACTICAL TIPS AND STRATEGIES FOR DAILY MANAGEMENT

Years ago, I had a patient named Martha who felt overwhelmed by her osteoporosis diagnosis. She struggled to find a way to manage her bone health effectively amidst her daily responsibilities. Her turning point came when she started setting clear, realistic goals. This approach transformed her outlook and empowered her to take control of her bone health. Martha's experience underscores the power of setting realistic goals to manage bone health effectively.

6.1 SETTING REALISTIC GOALS FOR BONE HEALTH

Setting realistic goals is a cornerstone of effective bone health management. Establishing clear objectives provides direction and focus, helping you prioritize what needs to be done to improve your bone health. It enhances your motivation and commitment, giving you a sense of purpose and a roadmap to follow. Moreover, setting goals allows you to measure your progress and celebrate your successes, which can be incredibly motivating.

When setting goals, it's crucial to use the SMART criteria. This framework ensures that your goals are Specific, Measurable, Achievable, Relevant, and Time-bound. Specific goals are clear and precise, avoiding vague statements. For example, instead of saying, "I want to improve my bone health," you might say, "I would like to increase my daily calcium intake by 300 milligrams." Measurable goals have quantifiable outcomes, allowing you to track your progress. Using the previous example, you can easily measure whether you've increased your calcium intake by checking your daily food diary or supplement log.

Achievable goals are realistic and attainable, considering your current health status and lifestyle. Setting a goal to run a marathon next month might not be feasible, but committing to a 30-minute walk three times a week is more realistic and still beneficial for bone health. Relevant goals are aligned with your overall health objectives. If your primary concern is preventing fractures, your goals should focus on activities and habits that directly impact bone strength and density. Finally, Time-bound goals have deadlines for completion, providing a sense of urgency and a timeline to work within. For instance, you might set a goal to schedule and attend a bone density scan within the next three months.

Let's explore some specific examples of realistic goals that can help you manage your bone health. One goal might be to increase your daily calcium intake by 300 milligrams. This can be achieved by incorporating more calcium-rich foods into your diet, such as dairy products, leafy greens, or fortified cereals, or by taking a calcium supplement if recommended by your healthcare provider. Another goal could be to complete a 30-minute exercise routine three times a week. This routine might include weight-bearing exercises like walking or dancing, combined with strength training exercises such as resistance band workouts or light weightlifting. A third example might be scheduling and attending a bone density scan within the next three months. This goal ensures that you are monitoring your bone health regularly and can make informed decisions based on the results.

Periodically reviewing and adjusting your goals is essential for continued progress. Monthly check-ins can help you assess how well you are meeting your goals and identify any barriers or challenges you might be facing. If you find that a particular goal is too ambitious or not yielding the desired results, don't hesitate to adjust it. Perhaps increasing your calcium intake by 300 milligrams daily is too challenging; you might scale back to 200 milligrams and gradually work your way up. Adjusting goals based on new health information, such as changes in your bone density results or new dietary recommendations, ensures that your objectives remain relevant and effective.

Celebrating your achievements and setting new milestones is also crucial for maintaining motivation. When you reach a goal, take the time to acknowledge your hard work and success. This celebration can be as simple as treating yourself to a favorite activity or sharing your accomplishment with friends and family. Recognizing your progress reinforces positive behaviors and encourages you to continue working towards your bone health goals. Once you achieve a goal, set a new one to keep challenging yourself and making progress. For example, after successfully completing a 30-minute exercise routine three times a week for several months, you might aim to extend your workouts to 45 minutes or add another day of exercise each week.

Interactive Element: Goal-Setting Worksheet

To help you set and track your bone health goals, consider using a goal-setting worksheet. This tool can guide you through the process of establishing SMART goals and provide a structured format for regular review and adjustment.

- Goal: [e.g., Increase daily calcium intake by 300 milligrams]
- Specific: What exactly do you want to achieve?
- Measurable: How will you measure your progress?
- Achievable: Is this goal realistic given your current situation?
- Relevant: How does this goal align with your overall health objectives?
- Time-bound: What is your deadline for achieving this goal?

By setting realistic, SMART goals and regularly reviewing and adjusting them, you can effectively manage your bone health and work towards a stronger, healthier future.

6.2 DAILY HABITS FOR STRONGER BONES

Incorporating bone-strengthening habits into your daily routine can significantly impact your overall bone health. These habits are not just beneficial for maintaining bone density, but also for enhancing your quality of life. One of the most effective habits is incorporating weight-bearing activities into your daily routines. Weight-bearing exercises, such as walking, jogging, dancing, and stair climbing, help stimulate bone formation. These activities force your bones to work against gravity, which strengthens them. Additionally, ensuring adequate intake of calcium and vitamin D is crucial. Calcium is the primary building block of your bones, while vitamin D aids in its absorption. Both nutrients are fundamental to maintaining bone density and preventing conditions like osteoporosis. Maintaining good posture throughout the day is another habit that supports bone health. Proper posture reduces strain on your spine and joints, which can help prevent fractures and other bone-related issues.

Making these habits part of your daily life is easier than it might seem. Start by taking a daily walk, which benefits your bones and boosts your cardiovascular health. If you have the option, incorporate stairs instead of elevators into your routine. Every step you take helps build stronger bones. Adding calcium-rich foods to every meal is another practical tip. Enjoy yogurt or milk with breakfast, add leafy greens like kale or spinach to your lunch, and include a serving of cheese or almonds with your dinner. Using reminders can help you remember to take your supplements regularly. Set alarms on your phone or place sticky notes in visible areas to prompt you to take your calcium and vitamin D supplements at the same time each day.

Staying hydrated is another key component of bone health. Water is vital for overall health, including the health of your bones. Hydration plays a crucial role in nutrient absorption. When you're well-hydrated, your body can absorb calcium and other essential nutrients more efficiently. Aim to drink at least eight glasses of water a day. If you struggle to drink enough water, try carrying a water bottle with you or setting hourly reminders to take a sip. Hydration also helps keep your joints lubricated, reducing the risk of injury during physical activity.

Here's a sample daily routine that incorporates these bone-healthy habits. In the morning, start your day with a 10-minute stretching and weight-bearing exercise session. Stretching helps improve flexibility and prepares your muscles and joints for the day ahead. Follow this with a brisk walk around your neighborhood or on a treadmill. For breakfast, enjoy a calcium-rich meal such as a bowl of fortified cereal with milk or a smoothie with yogurt and fruit. In the afternoon, have a calcium-rich snack like a handful of almonds or a serving of cheese. Make sure to stay hydrated by drinking water throughout the day. If you find it challenging to drink plain water, try adding a slice of lemon or cucumber for flavor. In the evening, dedicate a few minutes to relaxation exercises and posture improvement. Practice sitting and standing with your back straight and shoulders relaxed. Yoga or gentle stretching can also be beneficial for improving posture and reducing stress.

To help you incorporate these habits, consider using a daily checklist. This checklist can serve as a reminder and help you stay on track with your bone health goals. Here's an example of what your checklist might include: "Morning: 10-minute stretching and weight-bearing exercise; Breakfast: calcium-rich meal; Afternoon: calcium-rich snack and hydration; Evening: relaxation and posture exercises." By following this structured routine, you can ensure that you are consistently supporting your bone health.

Integrating these daily habits can make a significant difference in maintaining and improving your bone health. Consistency is key, and with a little effort, these habits can become a natural part of your daily routine. Remember, every small step you take towards better bone health contributes to a stronger, healthier future.

6.3 TRACKING YOUR PROGRESS: TOOLS AND TECHNIQUES

When I think back to my patient, Robert, I recall how he felt lost managing his bone health. He tried various exercises and diets but couldn't see any tangible results. It wasn't until he started tracking his progress that things began to change. Monitoring progress can significantly enhance bone health management by providing motivation and accountability. When you see how far you've come, it boosts your morale and keeps you committed to your health goals. Tracking also helps identify areas needing improvement, allowing you to adjust your strategies for better outcomes.

Various tools can help you effectively track your bone health. One of the simplest and most effective methods is maintaining a bone health journal. In this journal, you can record your daily activities, dietary intake, and any symptoms or challenges you encounter. This written record provides a tangible way to see your progress over time. Mobile apps for nutrition and exercise are also incredibly useful. These apps offer features like meal logging, exercise tracking, and even reminders to take your supplements. They can provide instant feedback and make it easier to stick to your routine. Wearable fitness trackers are another excellent tool. These devices monitor your physical activity, heart rate, and even sleep patterns. By providing real-time data, they can help you make immediate adjustments to your lifestyle.

In your tracking efforts, focus on key metrics to get a comprehensive view of your bone health. Start by monitoring your daily calcium and vitamin D intake. Ensure you're meeting your nutritional goals by recording everything you consume, including supplements. Tracking your weekly exercise routines and activities is equally important. Note the type of exercise, duration, and intensity. This information helps you see if you're getting enough weight-bearing and resistance exercises, essential for bone strength. Monthly progress in weight-bearing exercises should also be tracked. Look for improvements in your endurance, strength, and flexibility. This monthly check can help you adjust your exercise routines to keep them effective and challenging.

To help you get started, consider using tracking templates. A weekly exercise log template can be a simple table where you record each day's activities, the type of exercise, and the duration. This log can help you identify patterns and make necessary adjustments. A daily nutrition tracker can be a straightforward checklist where you note your intake of calcium-rich foods and vitamin D sources. This tracker ensures you're getting the nutrients you need for bone health. A monthly bone health assessment checklist can be an invaluable tool. This checklist can include questions about your physical activity, dietary habits, and any new symptoms or health changes. Regularly filling out this checklist helps you stay on top of your bone health and make informed decisions.

Interactive Element: Tracking Template Examples

To aid you in your tracking journey, here are some sample templates you can use:

- Weekly Exercise Log Template:
    - Day: [e.g., Monday]
    - Exercise Type: [e.g., Walking, Resistance Training]
    - Duration: [e.g., 30 minutes]
    - Intensity: [e.g., Moderate]
- Daily Nutrition Tracker:
    - Breakfast: [e.g., Yogurt, Fortified Cereal]
    - Lunch: [e.g., Spinach Salad, Grilled Chicken]
    - Dinner: [e.g., Steamed Broccoli, Almonds]
    - Supplements: [e.g., Calcium 500mg, Vitamin D 800 IU]
- Monthly Bone Health Assessment Checklist:
    - Physical Activity: [e.g., Increased/Decreased]
    - Dietary Habits: [e.g., Balanced/Needs Improvement]
    - Symptoms: [e.g., Joint Pain, Fatigue]

Using these templates, you can systematically track your progress, identify areas for improvement, and make informed decisions about your bone health. Tracking your progress keeps you accountable and provides a clear picture of your journey toward better bone health. Regular monitoring ensures that you stay on the right path and make necessary adjustments for optimal outcomes.

6.4 STAYING MOTIVATED: TIPS FOR CONSISTENCY

Maintaining motivation can be one of the most challenging aspects of managing your bone health. Several common obstacles often stand in the way. One of the main issues is the lack of immediate results. Unlike some health changes that show quick benefits, improvements in bone density and strength take time. This can make it difficult to stay motivated when you don't see noticeable changes right away. Physical discomfort or pain is another significant barrier. Exercise routines, especially if you're new to them, can lead to soreness or discomfort, making it tempting to skip sessions. Additionally, busy schedules and competing priorities can make it difficult to find the time and energy to focus on bone health. Life's daily demands often take precedence, leaving little room for consistent exercise and healthy eating.

To overcome these challenges, consider setting both short-term and long-term goals. Short-term goals provide immediate targets that are easier to achieve, keeping you motivated. For example, aiming to complete three exercise sessions in a week is a short-term goal that provides a quick sense of accomplishment. Long-term goals, such as improving your bone density over six months, give you something substantial to work towards. Finding a workout buddy can also be incredibly effective. Having someone to exercise with can provide accountability and make the experience more enjoyable. You can encourage each other on days when motivation is low. Rewarding yourself for reaching milestones is another excellent strategy. Small rewards, like enjoying a favorite treat or taking a relaxing bath, can make the effort feel more worthwhile and celebrate your progress.

Incorporating variety into your routine can keep things interesting and prevent boredom. Trying new exercises and activities can make your workouts more enjoyable. For instance, if you've been walking for exercise, you might try cycling or swimming to mix things up. Rotating different healthy recipes can also add excitement to your diet. Experiment with new ingredients and cooking methods to keep meals interesting and nutritious. Joining fitness classes or groups can provide both variety and social interaction. Being part of a group introduces you to new activities and offers a support network of like-minded individuals who share similar health goals.

Inspirational quotes and success stories can be powerful motivators. Hearing about others who have successfully improved their bone health can provide the encouragement you need to stay committed. For example, Jane, a senior who started with limited mobility, gradually built up her strength and now enjoys a more active lifestyle. Her story reminds us that progress is possible with perseverance. Health experts also offer valuable insights. Dr. Andrew Weil, a renowned expert in integrative medicine, once said, "The body has an astonishing capacity to heal itself. Our job is to support it through healthy choices." This quote emphasizes the importance of making consistent, healthy choices to support your bone health journey.

Textual Element: Reflection Section

Reflecting on your own experiences can also help maintain motivation. Take a moment to consider what has worked for you in the past and what challenges you've faced. Write down your thoughts and feelings about your progress and any obstacles you've encountered. This reflection can provide valuable insights and help you develop strategies to stay motivated.

Maintaining motivation is crucial for consistent bone health management. By setting both short-term and long-term goals, finding a workout buddy, and rewarding yourself for milestones, you can stay committed to your health. Incorporating variety in your routine and drawing inspiration from others can also keep things interesting and encourage you to stay on track. Reflecting on your journey and learning from your experiences can provide the insights needed to overcome challenges and continue making progress towards better bone health.

6.5 FALL PREVENTION: SAFE PRACTICES FOR HOME AND OUTDOORS

Preventing falls is critical for seniors, especially those with bone health issues like osteoporosis or arthritis. Falls can lead to fractures and other injuries, which can significantly impact your mobility and independence. By taking proactive steps to prevent falls, you can enhance your overall quality of life and maintain your independence longer. Reducing the risk of falls means you are less likely to experience the setbacks that can come with injuries, allowing you to continue engaging in the activities you enjoy.

Making your home safer is an essential step in fall prevention. Begin by installing grab bars in bathrooms, particularly near the toilet and in the shower or bathtub. These bars provide support and stability, reducing the risk of slipping or falling in wet areas. Removing tripping hazards is another crucial measure. Loose rugs, clutter, and electrical cords can easily cause trips and falls. Securing rugs with non-slip pads and keeping walkways clear can significantly reduce these risks. Ensuring adequate lighting throughout your home is also vital. Well-lit areas help you see potential obstacles and navigate your space safely. Consider adding nightlights in hallways and bathrooms to improve visibility during nighttime trips.

When you're outside the home, implementing safety practices is equally important. Wearing supportive footwear with good traction can help prevent slips and falls. Shoes with non-slip soles and proper arch support provide the stability needed for walking on various surfaces. Be cautious in wet or icy conditions, as these can be particularly hazardous. If the weather is bad, consider staying indoors or using pathways that have been cleared and treated. Carrying a walking aid, such as a cane or walker, can provide additional support and stability, especially if you have balance issues or are walking on uneven terrain.

Incorporating balance and stability exercises into your routine can also help reduce the risk of falls. Simple exercises like standing on one foot can significantly improve your balance. Start by standing near a sturdy surface, such as a countertop or chair, for support. Lift one foot off the ground and hold the position for 10 seconds, then switch to the other foot. Repeat this exercise several times a day to build balance and strength. The heel-to-toe walk is another effective exercise. Place one foot directly in front of the other, so the heel of your front foot touches the toes of your back foot. Walk forward in this manner for 20 steps, using a wall or railing for

PRACTICAL TIPS AND STRATEGIES FOR DAILY MANAGEMENT | 103

support if needed. This exercise helps improve coordination and stability.

Tai Chi is an excellent practice for enhancing balance and reducing fall risk. Tai Chi involves slow, deliberate movements that improve your balance, flexibility, and strength. Many seniors find Tai Chi beneficial because it is gentle on the joints and can be adapted to various fitness levels. Incorporating Tai Chi moves, such as the "Golden Rooster Stands on One Leg" or "Wave Hands Like Clouds," into your routine can provide significant balance benefits. Joining a local Tai Chi class or following along with instructional videos can help you get started and stay motivated.

Maintaining a safe environment and incorporating balance exercises are key strategies in fall prevention. By taking these proactive steps, you can significantly reduce your risk of falls and the associated injuries. This, in turn, allows you to maintain your independence and enjoy a higher quality of life. Whether you are making adjustments to your home, being cautious outdoors, or practicing balance exercises, each step you take towards preventing falls contributes to better bone health and overall well-being.

In the next chapter, we will explore the holistic health approach, integrating diet, exercise, and lifestyle changes to support comprehensive bone health. This approach will help you build a stronger foundation for long-term well-being.

7

HOLISTIC HEALTH APPROACH

Years ago, I had the pleasure of working with Irene, a spirited 70-year-old who loved dancing. She had a zest for life but struggled with bone density issues that threatened to curtail her passions. Irene's journey to better bone health was transformative when she embraced a holistic approach, integrating diet and exercise seamlessly into her daily routine. Her story serves as a powerful reminder that maintaining strong bones involves more than just one aspect of health; it requires a harmonious balance of nutrition and physical activity.

7.1 INTEGRATING DIET AND EXERCISE FOR BONE HEALTH

Combining proper nutrition with regular exercise is crucial for enhancing bone health. The synergy between these two elements creates a foundation for stronger bones and improved overall well-being. Nutrient absorption plays a significant role in muscle function, which is essential for supporting bone structure. When you engage in weight-bearing activities like walking or lifting weights, your body responds by increasing bone density. This process, known as bone remodeling, ensures that your bones remain resilient and less prone to fractures. On the other hand, a balanced diet rich in calcium, vitamin D, and other essential nutrients supports this process by providing the building blocks your body needs.

Timing your meals around workouts can optimize energy levels and enhance performance. Consuming a balanced meal that includes carbohydrates, proteins, and fats about two hours before exercising can provide the energy you need for a productive session. After your workout, focus on protein-rich snacks to aid in muscle recovery. Foods like Greek yogurt, nuts, or a protein shake can help repair muscle tissue and support bone health. By aligning your diet with your exercise routine, you create a powerful combination that maximizes the benefits of both.

Including protein-rich snacks post-exercise is particularly beneficial for muscle recovery. Protein helps repair and build muscle tissue, which in turn supports joint stability and reduces the risk of injuries. For instance, a post-workout smoothie made with Greek yogurt, berries, and a handful of spinach replenishes your energy and provides essential nutrients for bone health. This balanced approach ensures that your body gets the right fuel to recover and strengthen, making your bones more resilient over time.

The benefits of integrating diet and exercise extend beyond just bone health. This holistic approach enhances overall health and well-being, reducing the risk of chronic diseases such as diabetes and heart disease. Regular physical activity coupled with a nutritious diet helps maintain a healthy weight, improves cardiovascular health, and boosts mental well-being. For seniors, this balanced approach can lead to increased energy levels, better mobility, and a higher quality of life. By adopting these practices, you create a positive cycle where good nutrition fuels your exercise, and regular exercise enhances your overall health.

To illustrate this balanced approach, consider a sample daily plan. Start your day with a morning workout, such as a brisk walk or a gentle yoga session. Follow this with a post-exercise smoothie that includes Greek yogurt, berries, and a dash of honey for sweetness. This combination provides a good mix of protein, antioxidants, and natural sugars to kickstart your day. Midday, take a walk around your neighborhood or garden, and then enjoy a calcium-rich lunch, such as a spinach and salmon salad drizzled with lemon dressing. This meal not only supports bone health with calcium and vitamin D but also provides omega-3 fatty acids that reduce inflammation and support joint health.

By integrating these practices into your daily routine, you create a holistic approach to bone health that is effective and sustainable. This approach doesn't require drastic changes, but rather small, consistent adjustments that collectively make a significant difference. It's about making mindful choices that align with your body's needs and promoting overall well-being. Embracing this balanced approach ensures that you strengthen your bones and enhance your quality of life, allowing you to continue enjoying the activities you love.

7.2 STRESS MANAGEMENT TECHNIQUES FOR BETTER BONE HEALTH

Chronic stress can have a detrimental impact on bone health. When you're stressed, your body releases cortisol, a hormone that, in high levels, can lead to bone loss. Elevated cortisol levels accelerate bone resorption, where bone tissue is broken down, and the minerals are released into the bloodstream. This process weakens the bones over time, making them more susceptible to fractures. Stress also often leads to poor eating habits and inactivity, both of which negatively affect bone density. You might reach for comfort foods that lack essential nutrients or skip your regular exercises, further compromising your bone health.

Managing stress effectively is crucial for maintaining strong bones and overall health. One effective method is mindfulness meditation. This practice involves focusing on the present moment and accepting it without judgment. Mindfulness meditation can reduce stress by helping you develop a greater awareness of your thoughts and feelings, allowing you to respond to stressors more calmly. Deep breathing exercises are another simple yet powerful technique to manage stress. By taking slow, deep breaths, you can activate your body's relaxation response, which counteracts the stress response.

Progressive muscle relaxation is another method that can help reduce stress. This technique involves tensing and then slowly relaxing each muscle group in your body. It helps in releasing physical tension and can provide a sense of calm. Incorporating these stress management techniques into your daily routine can significantly improve your bone health. For example, setting aside just ten minutes a day for mindfulness meditation can make a noticeable difference. Practicing deep breathing exercises during breaks at work or while sitting in traffic can help keep stress levels in check.

To make these practices more effective, consider creating a dedicated space in your home for relaxation and meditation. This space can be as simple as a quiet corner with a comfortable chair and soft lighting. Consistency is key, so try to practice at the same time each day. You might find it helpful to start your day with a brief meditation session to set a calm tone, or end your day with progressive muscle relaxation to unwind before bed.

Reducing stress not only lowers cortisol levels but also has numerous other benefits for your health. Lower cortisol levels mean less bone loss and a reduced risk of osteoporosis. Additionally, managing stress can improve your overall mental and physical health. You'll likely experience better sleep, improved mood, and increased energy levels. These benefits create a positive feedback loop, where better health reduces stress, and reduced stress leads to better health. This holistic approach helps you maintain strong bones and enhances your quality of life.

7.3 SMOKING CESSATION AND BONE HEALTH

Smoking has a profoundly negative impact on bone health. It reduces calcium absorption, which is critical for maintaining bone density. Smoking also impairs blood flow to bones, depriving them of the oxygen and nutrients they need to stay strong. This combination of factors significantly increases the risk of fractures and slows down the healing process. Over time, the cumulative effect of smoking can lead to a significant loss of bone density, making bones brittle and more susceptible to breaks.

Quitting smoking can have immediate and long-term benefits for your bone health. Once you stop smoking, your body begins to repair the damage caused by tobacco. Improved circulation leads to better nutrient delivery to bones, which helps in maintaining and even increasing bone density over time. Additionally, quitting smoking reduces the risk of chronic diseases such as heart disease and cancer, further improving your overall health. This holistic improvement can enhance your quality of life and increase your lifespan.

Successfully quitting smoking often requires a multi-faceted approach. Behavioral therapy and support groups provide emotional and psychological support, helping you stay motivated and committed to quitting. Nicotine replacement therapy, such as patches or gum, can help manage withdrawal symptoms and reduce cravings. Prescription medications like varenicline and bupropion are also effective options that can aid in smoking cessation. These medications work by reducing cravings and withdrawal symptoms, making it easier to quit.

Hearing success stories from others who have quit smoking can be incredibly motivating. For example, Jane, a 65-year-old who smoked for over 30 years, decided to quit after being diagnosed with osteoporosis. Within a year of quitting, she noticed significant improvements in her bone density and overall health. Her energy levels increased, and she felt more capable of engaging in physical activities. Personal experiences like Jane's highlight the profound impact quitting smoking can have on bone health and overall well-being.

7.4 THE ROLE OF SLEEP IN BONE HEALTH

Quality sleep is crucial for maintaining bone health. During sleep, your body undergoes bone remodeling, a process where old bone tissue is broken down and new bone tissue is formed. This cycle is essential for keeping your bones strong and healthy. Adequate sleep also helps regulate hormones, including growth hormone, which plays a vital role in bone growth and repair. Without enough sleep, these processes are disrupted, leading to a decrease in bone density and an increased risk of osteoporosis.

Poor sleep has several negative effects on bone health. Inadequate sleep disrupts the balance between bone resorption and formation, making bones weaker and more susceptible to fractures. This disruption occurs because the lack of sleep interferes with the natural release of growth hormone and other regulatory hormones, impairing the body's ability to repair and build bone tissue. Additionally, poor sleep can impair nutrient absorption, meaning your body is less efficient at utilizing the vitamins and minerals necessary for bone health. Over time, these effects can lead to a significant reduction in bone density, increasing the risk of fractures and other bone-related issues.

Improving sleep quality can have a profound impact on your bone health. Establishing a regular sleep schedule is one of the most effective ways to ensure you get enough restful sleep. Going to bed and waking up at the same time every day helps regulate your body's internal clock, making it easier to fall asleep and stay asleep. Creating a sleep-conducive environment is also important. Make sure your bedroom is dark, quiet, and cool. Consider using blackout curtains to block out light, earplugs to minimize noise, or a white noise machine to create a soothing background sound. These adjustments can help you fall asleep faster and enjoy more restful sleep.

Avoiding caffeine and heavy meals before bedtime can also improve sleep quality. Caffeine is a stimulant that can keep you awake, so it's best to avoid it in the afternoon and evening. Heavy meals can cause discomfort and disrupt sleep, so try to have your last meal at least two to three hours before bedtime. Instead, opt for a light snack if you're hungry. Foods rich in tryptophan, such as turkey or bananas, can promote relaxation and help you sleep better.

Incorporating relaxation techniques into your bedtime routine can also promote better sleep. Reading a book, practicing gentle stretching, or listening to calming music can help you unwind and prepare for sleep. These activities signal to your body that it's time to relax and can make it easier to transition into sleep. Using sleep tracking apps can provide insights into your sleep patterns, helping you identify areas for improvement. These apps can track your sleep duration, quality, and cycles, giving you a clearer picture of your sleep health.

Interactive Element: Sleep Quality Checklist

- Establish a Regular Sleep Schedule: Go to bed and wake up at the same time every day.
- Create a Sleep-Conducive Environment: Ensure your bedroom is dark, quiet, and cool.
- Avoid Caffeine and Heavy Meals: Steer clear of caffeine in the afternoon and evening, and avoid heavy meals before bedtime.
- Incorporate Relaxation Techniques: Practice gentle stretching, read a book, or listen to calming music before bed.
- Use Sleep Tracking Apps: Monitor your sleep patterns to identify areas for improvement.

By following these tips and incorporating these practices into your routine, you can enhance your sleep quality and, in turn, improve your bone health. Quality sleep supports the essential processes of bone remodeling and hormonal regulation, ensuring that your bones remain strong and resilient.

7.5 REDUCING ALCOHOL INTAKE FOR STRONGER BONES

Excessive alcohol consumption can significantly harm your bone health. Alcohol interferes with calcium absorption, a critical mineral for maintaining bone density and strength. When you drink heavily, your digestive system struggles to absorb calcium efficiently, depriving your bones of the essential nutrients they need. This deficiency weakens your bones over time, making them more susceptible to fractures. Additionally, alcohol disrupts hormonal balances in your body. For instance, it can lower estrogen levels in women and testosterone levels in men, both of which play vital roles in maintaining bone density. These hormonal imbalances accelerate bone loss, further compromising bone strength.

Limiting alcohol intake offers numerous benefits for your bone health. One of the most immediate advantages is improved calcium absorption. By reducing alcohol consumption, your digestive system can better absorb calcium, which in turn strengthens your bones. Enhanced bone strength reduces the risk of fractures and other bone-related issues. Moreover, cutting down on alcohol can improve your overall health, reducing the risk of chronic diseases such as liver disease, heart disease, and certain cancers. This holistic improvement in health supports better bone density and enhances your quality of life.

To effectively reduce alcohol consumption, consider setting clear limits and tracking your intake. Keeping a journal of your drinking habits can provide valuable insights into patterns and help you identify triggers that lead to excessive drinking. Setting specific goals, such as limiting yourself to one drink per day or designating alcohol-free days each week, can make it easier to cut down. Finding alternative social activities that don't involve alcohol can also be beneficial. Instead of meeting friends at a bar, suggest activities like hiking, attending a fitness class, or visiting a museum. These alternatives not only help you reduce alcohol intake but also promote a more active and healthier lifestyle.

Support from friends, family, or support groups can make a significant difference in reducing alcohol consumption. Openly discussing your goals with loved ones can provide accountability and encouragement. Support groups, either in-person or online, offer a community of individuals with similar goals, providing mutual support and practical advice. These groups can be particularly helpful in navigating challenges and staying committed to your goals.

Exploring alcohol-free alternatives can make the transition easier and more enjoyable. Mocktails, or non-alcoholic cocktails, are a great way to enjoy flavorful and festive beverages without the negative effects of alcohol. Recipes for mocktails often include fresh fruits, herbs, and sparkling water, making them both delicious and nutritious. For example, a refreshing mocktail could include muddled mint leaves, lime juice, a splash of pomegranate juice, and sparkling water. Engaging in hobbies or physical activities can also serve as excellent distractions from drinking. Whether it's gardening, painting, or joining a local walking club, finding activities that you enjoy can help you stay focused on your goal of reducing alcohol intake.

Incorporating these strategies into your daily life can lead to significant improvements in both bone health and overall well-being. By understanding the impact of alcohol on your bones and taking proactive steps to reduce consumption, you can protect yourself from fractures and other bone-related issues. Limiting alcohol also contributes to better digestion, hormonal balance, and overall health, making it a worthwhile endeavor for anyone looking to improve their quality of life.

In the next chapter, we'll explore practical tips and strategies for daily bone health management, including setting realistic goals, tracking progress, and staying motivated. These insights will help you maintain and improve your bone health, ensuring a more active and fulfilling life.

8

PERSONAL STORIES AND TESTIMONIALS

8.1 OVERCOMING OSTEOPOROSIS: JANE'S STORY

Jane's journey began with an unsettling diagnosis that turned her world upside down. At the age of 50, she was diagnosed with severe osteoporosis, a condition that left her bones brittle and vulnerable to fractures. The news hit Jane like a ton of bricks. She had always been active, enjoying brisk walks and participating in community events. The diagnosis filled her with fear and uncertainty. She worried about her future and how this condition would impact her daily life. The term "osteoporosis" was foreign to her, and she felt overwhelmed by the lack of knowledge she had about managing it.

Determined not to let osteoporosis control her life, Jane took proactive steps to manage her condition. She began by consulting her healthcare provider to create a personalized treatment plan. Her doctor explained the importance of a multifaceted approach, combining medication, supplements, and lifestyle changes. Jane started a regimen of calcium and vitamin D supplements to support her bone health. Calcium is vital for bone formation and maintenance, while vitamin D enhances calcium absorption, ensuring that her bones received the necessary nutrients. Jane's commitment to her supplement routine was unwavering, as she understood that this was a crucial part of her treatment.

Jane also incorporated specific exercises into her daily routine to strengthen her bones and improve her overall health. She began with weight-bearing exercises like walking and light jogging. These activities helped stimulate bone formation and increased her bone density over time. Jane also added strength training to her regimen, using resistance bands to build muscle and support her skeletal system. She found that these exercises not only helped her bones but also improved her balance and coordination, reducing her risk of falls. Jane's dedication to her exercise routine was evident as she diligently followed her plan, gradually increasing the intensity and duration of her workouts.

The results of Jane's efforts were nothing short of remarkable. After a year of sticking to her treatment plan and exercise routine, Jane saw a significant improvement in her bone density. Her follow-up bone density scans showed that her bones had become stronger, and her risk of fractures had decreased. Jane also noticed an increase in her energy levels and overall well-being. She felt more confident in her ability to stay active and engaged in her community. Jane's success story is a testament to the power of a well-rounded approach to managing osteoporosis.

Jane's advice to others facing a similar diagnosis is simple yet profound. She encourages you to take an active role in managing your bone health. Consulting with healthcare providers is essential to create a personalized plan that addresses your specific needs. Jane emphasizes the importance of sticking to a supplement regimen and incorporating weight-bearing and strength-training exercises into your daily routine. She believes that maintaining a positive attitude and staying committed to your plan can make a world of difference. Jane's story serves as an inspiration, showing that with determination and the right strategies, you can overcome the challenges of osteoporosis and lead a fulfilling life.

8.2 FROM DIAGNOSIS TO RECOVERY: MARK'S JOURNEY

Mark's struggles began long before his diagnosis. As a 68-year-old retired engineer, he enjoyed woodworking and hiking. However, he started experiencing frequent fractures and persistent bone pain. Simple tasks became challenging. Opening jars, lifting light objects, and even standing for extended periods caused discomfort. His morning routine, once filled with vigor, turned into a series of small battles against pain and weakness. These difficulties were not just physical; they weighed heavily on his spirit. He felt frustrated and helpless, unsure of the cause behind his declining health.

When Mark was diagnosed with severe osteoporosis, it was both a shock and a relief. The diagnosis provided an explanation for his struggles, but it also introduced new fears. He was determined not to let osteoporosis define him. Mark decided to take a proactive approach to his health. He consulted his healthcare provider to develop a comprehensive treatment plan. His doctor explained the importance of addressing the condition from multiple angles, combining medication, diet, and physical therapy. Mark was committed to making the necessary changes to improve his bone health.

Mark's treatment plan was multifaceted, reflecting his determination to tackle osteoporosis head-on. His doctor prescribed medications designed to improve bone density. These included bisphosphonates, which slow down bone loss and help build bone mass. Mark also made significant nutritional changes. He incorporated more calcium-rich foods into his diet, such as dairy products and leafy greens. Vitamin D supplements became a regular part of his routine, ensuring that his body could efficiently absorb calcium. Mark's commitment to these dietary adjustments was unwavering, as he understood their critical role in supporting his bones.

Regular physical therapy sessions became another cornerstone of Mark's treatment plan. He worked with a skilled physical therapist who tailored exercises to his specific needs. These sessions included weight-bearing activities, such as walking and light jogging, to stimulate bone growth. Strength training exercises using resistance bands and light weights helped build muscle and support his skeletal system. Mark also incorporated balance exercises to reduce his risk of falls. The physical therapy sessions not only improved his bone density but also enhanced his overall mobility and confidence.

Mark's recovery was nothing short of remarkable. Over time, he noticed a significant improvement in his bone density. His follow-up scans showed that his bones had become stronger, and the frequency of fractures decreased. Mark's pain levels diminished, allowing him to return to his favorite activities like hiking. He found joy in the simple pleasures of life, like taking long walks in nature and working on his woodworking projects. The improvement in his physical health also boosted his mental well-being. He felt more energetic and optimistic about his future.

Mark's advice to others facing similar challenges is straightforward and heartfelt. He emphasizes the importance of staying positive and persistent. Managing osteoporosis is a long-term commitment, but the results are worth the effort. He encourages you to work closely with healthcare professionals to develop a personalized treatment plan. Mark believes in the power of combining medication, nutrition, and physical therapy to achieve the best outcomes. He also stresses the importance of regular check-ups and bone density scans to monitor progress and make necessary adjustments. Mark's journey is a testament to the power of determination and a well-rounded approach to managing osteoporosis.

8.3 STAYING ACTIVE WITH ARTHRITIS: LINDA'S EXPERIENCE

Linda's journey with arthritis began with persistent, debilitating joint pain and stiffness. Every morning, she struggled to get out of bed, her joints creaking and aching with every movement. Simple tasks, like opening a jar or walking to the mailbox, became daunting challenges. The stiffness in her knees and hips limited her mobility, making daily activities nearly impossible without pain. Linda felt trapped in her own body, her once-active life reduced to a series of cautious, painful steps. The prospect of maintaining any physical activity seemed distant, and the fear of aggravating her condition loomed large.

Determined not to let arthritis dictate her life, Linda sought ways to stay active that would accommodate her condition. She discovered that low-impact exercises were the key to managing her arthritis while staying physically engaged. Swimming became her sanctuary. The buoyancy of the water alleviated the pressure on her joints, allowing her to move freely without pain. She joined a local water aerobics class, where she found both physical relief and a supportive community. The gentle resistance of the water helped strengthen her muscles and improve her flexibility without straining her joints.

In addition to her aquatic activities, Linda incorporated gentle yoga and stretching routines into her daily regimen. These exercises helped maintain her joint flexibility and reduce stiffness. Poses like the child's pose, cat-cow stretch, and gentle twists became staples of her routine. She also practiced deep breathing exercises, which enhanced her flexibility and helped manage her stress levels. The combination of physical movement and mindfulness provided Linda with a holistic approach to managing her arthritis. She felt a renewed sense of control over her body and her condition.

The improvements Linda experienced were profound. Over time, her chronic joint pain diminished, and her flexibility increased. She found that she could participate in community activities and social events that she had previously avoided due to her pain. Linda began attending local gardening clubs, where she could engage in light gardening tasks without discomfort. She also joined a book club, enjoying the camaraderie and discussions with fellow members. These activities enriched her life, giving her a sense of purpose and connection. The physical improvements also boosted her mental well-being, as she felt more confident and capable.

Linda's advice to others facing similar challenges with arthritis is both practical and encouraging. She emphasizes the importance of finding activities that you enjoy and that suit your condition. Whether it's swimming, yoga, or any other low impact exercise, the key is to stay active in a way that feels good for your body. Consistency is crucial. Linda found that sticking to her exercise routine, even on days when she felt less motivated, made a significant difference in managing her pain and maintaining her mobility. She also encourages seeking support from friends and family. Having a workout buddy or someone to share your journey with can provide motivation and make the experience more enjoyable.

Linda's story is a testament to the power of perseverance and finding the right balance to live a fulfilling life with arthritis.

8.4 THE POWER OF NUTRITION: RACHEL'S TRANSFORMATION

Rachel's health journey began with frequent bone pain and persistent weakness that hampered her daily activities. As a 62-year-old retiree who had always enjoyed gardening and spending time with her grandchildren, Rachel found herself increasingly limited by her deteriorating bone health. Her diet was a significant contributing factor. She often relied on convenience foods, which lacked the nutrients necessary for maintaining strong bones. Her meals were deficient in calcium, vitamin D, and other vital nutrients, exacerbating her condition. Rachel's initial understanding of bone health was minimal, and she felt overwhelmed by the changes she needed to make.

Determined to improve her health, Rachel decided to overhaul her diet. The first step was incorporating more calcium-rich foods into her meals. She started including dairy products like milk, cheese, and yogurt in her daily diet. These foods provided a substantial boost in calcium intake, which is crucial for bone strength. Rachel also discovered the benefits of leafy green vegetables such as kale, spinach, and broccoli. These vegetables became a staple in her meals, offering not only calcium but also other essential nutrients that support bone health. She added these greens to her salads, smoothies, and side dishes, ensuring a consistent intake of calcium.

In addition to calcium, Rachel understood the importance of vitamin D for bone health. Vitamin D facilitates calcium absorption, making it essential for maintaining strong bones. She began incorporating vitamin D-rich foods into her diet, such as fatty fish like salmon and mackerel. These fish not only provided vitamin D but also omega-3 fatty acids, which have anti-inflammatory properties beneficial for overall health. Rachel also included fortified cereals and orange juice in her breakfast routine, further enhancing her vitamin D intake. To address any potential deficiencies, she started taking vitamin D supplements under her healthcare provider's guidance, ensuring she met her daily requirements.

Rachel's commitment to improving her diet extended to addressing potential nutritional gaps through supplements. In addition to vitamin D, she began taking magnesium and vitamin K2 supplements. Magnesium plays a crucial role in bone formation and helps convert vitamin D into its active form, while vitamin K2 directs calcium to the bones, preventing it from depositing in the arteries. These supplements complemented her dietary changes, providing a comprehensive approach to bone health. Rachel's careful attention to her nutritional needs made a significant difference in her overall well-being.

The transformation Rachel experienced was remarkable. Over time, she noticed a substantial increase in her bone density, as confirmed by her follow-up bone density scans. The frequent bone pain and weakness that once plagued her daily life diminished significantly. Rachel felt more energetic and capable of engaging in activities she had previously avoided. Gardening, which had become a painful task, once again became a source of joy and relaxation. She found herself able to spend more time with her grandchildren, participating in their games and activities without the constant fear of pain or injury. Rachel's overall health improved, and she felt more vibrant and active than she had in years.

Rachel's advice for others looking to improve their bone health through nutrition is both practical and insightful. She emphasizes the importance of a balanced diet that includes a diverse range of nutrients. Ensuring that your meals are rich in calcium and vitamin D is crucial, but it's also essential to include other nutrients like magnesium and vitamin K2. Rachel recommends planning meals ahead of time to ensure a consistent intake of these nutrients. She found that preparing a weekly meal plan and grocery list helped her stay on track and avoid the temptation of convenience foods. Rachel also advises staying informed about your nutritional needs and being open to adjustments as necessary. Consulting with healthcare providers and nutritionists can provide valuable guidance tailored to your specific health requirements.

Rachel's story is a powerful testament to the impact of nutrition on bone health. Her dedication to improving her diet and addressing nutritional gaps through supplements led to significant improvements in her bone density and overall well-being. By following her advice and committing to a balanced diet, you too can enhance your bone health and enjoy a more active and fulfilling life.

8.5 HOLISTIC HEALTH SUCCESS: JOHN'S TESTIMONY

John's story is one of unwavering commitment to a holistic approach to managing his bone health. At 65, John faced the unsettling news of declining bone density. Rather than feeling defeated, he embraced a comprehensive strategy that integrated diet, exercise, stress management, and sleep. His determination to find a balanced approach was evident from the start. John believed that addressing bone health required more than just medication; it needed a lifestyle overhaul. He was not content with just taking pills; he wanted to transform how he lived each day to ensure better bone health and overall well-being.

John's comprehensive plan involved several specific strategies. He started with regular weight-bearing and resistance exercises. Understanding that movement is vital for bone strength, John incorporated activities like walking, hiking, and light jogging into his routine. He also added resistance training using weights and resistance bands to build muscle and support his skeletal system. These exercises not only helped improve his bone density but also enhanced his overall fitness and stamina. John committed to these activities daily, gradually increasing intensity and duration as his strength improved.

Equally important was his focus on a balanced diet rich in bone-healthy nutrients. John made significant changes to his eating habits, ensuring that every meal contributed to his bone health. He included ample sources of calcium, such as dairy products, leafy greens, and fortified foods. Understanding the role of vitamin D in calcium absorption, he added vitamin D-rich foods like fatty fish and fortified cereals to his diet. John also took magnesium and vitamin K2 supplements to ensure that his bones received all the necessary nutrients. His meals were carefully planned and prepared, emphasizing whole foods and minimizing processed items.

Stress management became another cornerstone of John's holistic approach. He recognized that chronic stress could negatively impact bone health by increasing cortisol levels, which can lead to bone loss. To counter this, John adopted mindfulness meditation and deep breathing exercises. He set aside time each day to practice these techniques, which helped him stay calm and centered. These practices not only reduced his stress levels but also improved his mental clarity and emotional resilience. John found that managing stress was as crucial as physical exercise in maintaining his overall health.

Prioritizing quality sleep was another essential element of John's plan. He understood that adequate sleep is vital for bone remodeling and repair. John established a consistent sleep routine, going to bed and waking up at the same time each day. He created a sleep-conducive environment by keeping his bedroom dark, quiet, and cool. Avoiding caffeine and heavy meals before bedtime helped him fall asleep more easily and enjoy a deeper rest. Over time, these changes significantly improved the quality of his sleep, which in turn supported his bone health.

The outcomes of John's holistic approach were remarkable. His bone density saw significant improvement, as confirmed by follow-up scans. The strength he gained from regular exercise allowed him to maintain an active lifestyle, participating in activities he loved without fear of injury. His mental and physical well-being flourished, with reduced stress levels and enhanced energy. John felt more vibrant and capable, enjoying a fulfilling life that balanced all aspects of his health. He found joy in the process and satisfaction in seeing the positive changes in his body and mind.

John's advice for others considering a holistic approach to bone health is rooted in his own experiences. He emphasizes the importance of a balanced and integrated approach, combining diet, exercise, stress management, and sleep. Consistency and patience are key. John believes that small, daily actions lead to significant long-term benefits. He encourages finding joy and satisfaction in the journey toward better health, celebrating each milestone along the way. John's story is a powerful example of how a comprehensive, holistic approach can lead to remarkable improvements in bone health and overall well-being.

9

ADDRESSING COMMON PAIN POINTS AND QUESTIONS

Years ago, I remember a patient named Evelyn who had always been a pillar of her community. She was known for her vibrant spirit and active participation in local events. However, after a series of minor falls, Evelyn began to withdraw from her social activities. She confided in me that her fear of falling had become overwhelming. This fear is not uncommon among seniors and highlights the critical importance of fall prevention for those with bone health issues.

9.1 SAFE EXERCISES TO PREVENT FALLS

Preventing falls is a cornerstone of maintaining bone health and overall well-being as we age. Falls are the leading cause of injuries among older adults, often resulting in fractures that can drastically reduce mobility and independence. By reducing the risk of falls, you can significantly enhance your quality of life, minimize hospital visits, and avoid the associated healthcare costs. Each fall prevented is a step towards maintaining your autonomy and continuing to enjoy the activities you love.

Improving balance and stability through targeted exercises is an effective way to prevent falls. One simple but powerful exercise is the single leg stand. Stand near a sturdy chair or counter for support, lift one foot off the ground, and try to balance on the other leg for 10 seconds. Repeat this exercise on the other leg. This exercise strengthens the muscles in your legs and improves your overall balance. Another effective exercise is the heel-to-toe walk. Imagine you are walking on a tightrope, placing the heel of one foot directly in front of the toes of the other foot. Walk this way for about 20 steps. This exercise challenges your balance and coordination, making you more stable on your feet. Side leg raises are also beneficial. Stand with your feet shoulder-width apart, lift one leg out to the side, and lower it back down slowly. Perform 2 sets of 10 repetitions on each leg. This exercise strengthens the muscles around your hips, which are crucial for maintaining balance.

Environmental modifications can also play a significant role in reducing fall risk. Start by removing tripping hazards such as loose rugs and clutter from your home. These items can easily cause you to trip and fall, especially in low-light conditions. Installing grab bars in bathrooms and along staircases provides additional support where it is most needed. Grab bars offer a stable handhold, making it easier to navigate tricky areas. Ensuring adequate lighting in all areas of your home, especially stairways and hallways, is essential. Good lighting helps you see obstacles clearly and reduces the risk of tripping. Consider using night lights or motion-sensor lights to illuminate your path during the night.

When exercising, it is crucial to follow safe practices to prevent falls. Always wear supportive footwear with good traction. Proper shoes can provide stability and reduce the risk of slipping. Ensure you are exercising on even surfaces to avoid unexpected trips and falls. Having a sturdy chair or railing nearby for support is also a good idea, especially when trying new exercises or if your balance is not yet strong. This support can prevent falls and give you the confidence to push yourself a little further.

Incorporating these exercises and environmental changes into your daily routine can significantly reduce your risk of falling. Remember, the goal is to improve your stability and confidence, allowing you to move freely and continue enjoying your favorite activities without fear. Fall prevention is not just about avoiding injuries; it's about maintaining your independence and quality of life. By taking these proactive steps, you can create a safer environment and build a stronger, more stable body.

9.2 NAVIGATING NUTRITIONAL NEEDS WITHOUT CONFUSION

Understanding the nutrients essential for bone health is the first step toward maintaining strong bones. Calcium is vital as it forms the building blocks of your bones. Aim to include calcium-rich foods in your diet, such as dairy products, leafy green vegetables, and fortified plant-based milks. Vitamin D is equally important because it enhances your body's ability to absorb calcium. You can get vitamin D from sunlight, fatty fish like salmon, and fortified foods. Magnesium plays a crucial role in bone formation and maintenance, and it can be found in nuts, seeds, and whole grains. Vitamin K2 helps direct calcium to your bones and away from arteries, reducing the risk of arterial calcification. You can find Vitamin K2 in fermented foods and certain cheeses. Lastly, protein is essential for muscle support and overall health, which in turn helps maintain bone strength. Include sources like lean meats, beans, and legumes in your diet.

Creating balanced meals doesn't have to be complicated. A simple guide is to divide your plate into sections: half of it should be filled with vegetables, a quarter with protein, and the remaining quarter with whole grains. This approach ensures you're getting various nutrients in each meal. Make it a habit to include a calcium-rich food in every meal—think of adding a slice of cheese to your breakfast, a yogurt cup with lunch, or a serving of broccoli with dinner. To enhance flavor without adding sodium, use herbs and spices. Fresh herbs like basil, rosemary, and cilantro can elevate the taste of your dishes without the need for extra salt.

There are many myths about nutrition and bone health that can lead to confusion. One common misconception is that only dairy products provide enough calcium. While dairy is a rich source, many non-dairy foods are also high in calcium. Almonds, tofu, and fortified orange juice are excellent examples. Another myth is that high-protein diets are bad for bones. This belief stems from the idea that protein increases calcium excretion. However, recent studies suggest that a moderate increase in dietary protein can actually benefit bone health by enhancing calcium absorption and increasing muscle mass. Protein from both animal and plant sources can contribute to maintaining strong bones.

Planning bone-healthy meals is easier when you approach it with a strategy. Start by creating weekly meal plans and grocery lists. This preparation ensures you have all the ingredients needed for balanced meals and prevents last-minute unhealthy choices. Batch cooking and freezing meals can save time and make it easier to stick to your nutritional goals. Prepare large batches of soups, stews, or casseroles, and freeze portions for later use. Trying new recipes can keep your meals interesting and nutritious. Experiment with different cuisines and cooking methods to find what you enjoy. For example, you might try a new way of preparing salmon with a side of quinoa and steamed vegetables, or a hearty lentil soup with a fresh herb salad.

Interactive Element: Weekly Meal Planning Template

Create a meal plan for the week, including breakfast, lunch, dinner, and snacks. List the ingredients needed for each meal and prepare a grocery list. Example:

- Monday:
    - Breakfast: Greek yogurt with berries and almonds
    - Lunch: Spinach and salmon salad with lemon dressing
    - Dinner: Grilled chicken with quinoa and steamed broccoli
    - Snack: Cottage cheese with pineapple

Navigating the landscape of nutritional needs doesn't have to be overwhelming. By understanding the key nutrients necessary for bone health, debunking common myths, and incorporating practical meal planning tips, you can create a diet that supports strong bones and overall well-being. Balancing your plate, trying new recipes, and planning ahead can make a significant difference in maintaining your bone density and strength as you age.

9.3 MANAGING LIMITED MOBILITY IN EXERCISE ROUTINES

Physical limitations can pose significant challenges when trying to maintain an exercise routine. Joint pain and stiffness often make movement difficult, and reduced range of motion can limit the types of exercises you can perform. Additionally, the fear of injury or exacerbating existing conditions can deter you from staying active. Recognizing these difficulties is the first step toward finding effective solutions. It's crucial to understand that even with limited mobility, you can still engage in exercises that benefit your bone health and overall well-being.

Modified exercises can be incredibly effective for those with limited mobility. Seated leg lifts, for example, allow you to work on your lower body strength without putting undue pressure on your joints. Sit tall in a sturdy chair, lift one leg straight out, hold it for a few seconds, and then lower it. Repeat this for 2 sets of 10 repetitions per leg. Arm circles while seated are another excellent option. Sit upright, extend your arms to the sides, and make small circular motions. Perform 2 sets of 15 repetitions. This exercise helps maintain shoulder flexibility and strengthens your upper body. Seated marches are also beneficial. Sit on the edge of a chair, lift your knees alternately as if you were marching. Complete 2 sets of 10 repetitions per leg. These exercises can be done in the comfort of your own home and require minimal equipment.

Adaptive equipment can further assist in performing exercises safely and effectively. Resistance bands are versatile tools that can add an extra level of challenge to your seated strength training. They come in various resistance levels, allowing you to start light and gradually increase the difficulty. Stability balls can be used for supported exercises that improve balance and core strength. Sitting on a stability ball while performing arm exercises, for example, engages your core muscles and enhances stability. Hand weights are excellent for upper body strength training. They are available in various weights, so you can choose the one that suits your current strength level. Using these tools can make your exercise routine more effective and enjoyable.

Staying active despite mobility challenges requires some practical adjustments. Breaking exercise sessions into shorter, more manageable segments can make it easier to stick with your routine. Instead of aiming for a 30-minute session, try three 10-minute sessions spread throughout the day. Incorporating movement into your daily activities can also help. Stretch while watching TV, do a few leg lifts during commercial breaks, or take a short walk around your home. Finding low-impact activities like swimming or water aerobics can be beneficial. The buoyancy of water reduces the strain on your joints while still providing a good workout. Many community centers offer classes designed specifically for seniors, making it easier to find activities that suit your needs and preferences.

Adaptive equipment can further assist in performing exercises safely and effectively. Resistance bands are versatile tools that can add an extra level of challenge to your seated strength training. They come in various resistance levels, allowing you to start light and gradually increase the difficulty. Stability balls can be used for supported exercises that improve balance and core strength. Sitting on a stability ball while performing arm exercises, for example, engages your core muscles and enhances stability. Hand weights are excellent for upper body strength training. They are available in various weights, so you can choose the one that suits your current strength level. Using these tools can make your exercise routine more effective and enjoyable.

Staying active despite mobility challenges requires some practical adjustments. Breaking exercise sessions into shorter, more manageable segments can make it easier to stick with your routine. Instead of aiming for a 30-minute session, try three 10-minute sessions spread throughout the day. Incorporating movement into your daily activities can also help. Stretch while watching TV, do a few leg lifts during commercial breaks, or take a short walk around your home. Finding low-impact activities like swimming or water aerobics can be beneficial. The buoyancy of water reduces the strain on your joints while still providing a good workout. Many community centers offer classes designed specifically for seniors, making it easier to find activities that suit your needs and preferences.

9.4 EFFECTIVE SUPPLEMENTATION: WHAT ACTUALLY WORKS

Supplements play a crucial role in maintaining bone health, especially for those who may not get all the necessary nutrients from their diet. They help fill nutritional gaps, supporting bone density and overall strength. Adequate supplementation can significantly enhance your well-being by ensuring that your bones receive the nutrients they need to stay strong and resilient. Supplements are particularly vital for seniors who may have decreased nutrient absorption or dietary restrictions.

Evidence-based supplements have proven effective in supporting bone health. Calcium is fundamental for bone formation and maintenance. Ensuring that you get the recommended daily intake, which is 1,000 mg for those 50 and younger and 1,200 mg for those over 50, helps maintain bone density. Vitamin D is equally important, as it aids in the absorption of calcium. You need between 800 and 1,000 IU of vitamin D daily to ensure that the calcium you consume is effectively utilized by your body. Magnesium, another essential mineral, supports bone formation and maintenance. It acts as a co-factor in many enzymatic reactions that contribute to bone health. The recommended daily intake for magnesium ranges from 310 to 420 mg, depending on age and gender. Vitamin K2 is also beneficial as it helps direct calcium to your bones and away from your arteries, reducing the risk of arterial calcification and promoting better bone density.

Choosing high-quality supplements requires careful consideration. Look for products that have undergone third-party testing and certifications to ensure their quality and potency. Reputable brands often display these certifications on their labels. Avoid supplements with unnecessary additives and fillers that do not contribute to your health. These can include artificial colors, flavors, and preservatives. Instead, opt for supplements with fewer ingredients and focus on the active components. Selecting appropriate dosages based on your individual needs is also crucial. Consult your healthcare provider to determine the correct dosages for your specific situation. They can provide personalized recommendations based on your health status, dietary intake, and any medications you may be taking.

Common concerns about supplementation often revolve around potential side effects. For instance, calcium supplements can cause gastrointestinal issues such as constipation, bloating, or gas. To mitigate these side effects, consider taking calcium supplements with meals and increasing your water and fiber intake. If you experience persistent discomfort, switching to a different form of calcium, such as calcium citrate, which is easier on the stomach, might help. Vitamin D toxicity is another concern, particularly if taken in excessive amounts. Symptoms of vitamin D toxicity include nausea, vomiting, weakness, and kidney problems. To avoid this, stick to the recommended dosages and have your blood levels monitored regularly by your healthcare provider. They can adjust your dosage if necessary to ensure you are within safe limits.

Supplements can be a valuable addition to your bone health regimen, especially when dietary intake alone is insufficient. They provide a reliable way to ensure that your bones receive the nutrients they need to remain strong and healthy. Always choose high-quality products, consult your healthcare provider for personalized advice, and be mindful of potential side effects to make the most of your supplementation strategy.

9.5 STAYING CONSISTENT: OVERCOMING MOTIVATION BARRIERS

Maintaining a consistent bone health routine can be challenging, especially when faced with common motivation barriers. One significant obstacle is the lack of immediate results. When you start a new exercise or dietary regimen, it can take weeks or even months to see tangible improvements in bone density or reduced pain. This delayed gratification often leads to frustration and discouragement. You might feel like your efforts are in vain, especially when the progress isn't visible right away. Additionally, physical discomfort or pain can make it difficult to stay committed. If exercises cause joint pain or muscle soreness, you may be tempted to skip sessions or abandon the routine altogether. Busy schedules and competing priorities also pose significant hurdles. With numerous responsibilities, finding time for exercise and meal planning can seem overwhelming, leading to inconsistent adherence.

To overcome these barriers, setting both short-term and long-term goals can be immensely helpful. Short-term goals provide immediate targets to strive for, such as completing a week's worth of exercise sessions or incorporating more calcium-rich foods into your diet. These smaller milestones can offer a sense of accomplishment and keep you motivated. Long-term goals, like improving bone density or reducing the risk of fractures, give you a broader vision to work towards. Keeping a progress journal can also be beneficial. Document your daily activities, noting any improvements or setbacks. This journal serves as a tangible record of your journey, allowing you to track progress over time and adjust your strategies as needed. Rewarding yourself for reaching milestones is another effective strategy. Treat yourself to a small reward, like a new book or a special outing, when you achieve a goal. These rewards provide positive reinforcement and can make the process more enjoyable.

Support systems play a crucial role in maintaining motivation. Finding a workout buddy can provide accountability and make exercise sessions more enjoyable. You can encourage each other, share tips, and celebrate achievements together. Joining fitness classes or groups offers social interaction and a sense of community. Being part of a group with similar goals can provide additional motivation and make the experience more engaging. Seeking encouragement from friends and family is equally important. Share your goals with them and ask for their support. They can offer words of encouragement, join you in activities, or help keep you accountable.

Inspirational quotes and stories can also serve as powerful motivators. Hearing from seniors who have successfully maintained a bone-health routine can provide hope and encouragement. For example, Linda, a 70-year-old, shared her story of overcoming arthritis pain through consistent exercise and dietary changes. Her dedication led to significant improvements in her mobility and overall well-being. Quotes from health experts and motivational speakers can also provide a boost. One such quote is, "The only limit to our realization of tomorrow is our doubts of today," reminding us that perseverance and belief in our abilities can lead to remarkable outcomes.

Incorporating these strategies and seeking support can help you overcome motivation barriers and stay consistent in your bone health routine. The journey may have its challenges, but with determination and the right support, you can make meaningful progress.

In the next chapter, we will explore practical tools and interactive elements to further assist you in your bone health journey. These tools are designed to keep you engaged, provide structure, and enhance your overall experience. From exercise tracking charts to supplement dosage schedules, you'll find valuable resources to help you stay on track and achieve your bone health goals.

10

INTERACTIVE ELEMENTS AND TOOLS

When I met Louise, she was a diligent 70-year-old eager to regain her strength after a hip fracture. She found herself overwhelmed by the variety of exercises and unsure how to track her progress. Louise's experience inspired me to emphasize the importance of exercise tracking charts. These tools can transform your approach to fitness by providing a clear roadmap and helping you visualize your progress. Tracking your exercise routines can be a game-changer, offering both accountability and motivation.

10.1 EXERCISE TRACKING CHARTS

Exercise tracking charts serve as a powerful tool to monitor your fitness routines. They offer a visual representation of your progress, which can be incredibly motivating. Seeing your efforts laid out on paper or a digital platform helps identify patterns and areas needing improvement. For instance, you might notice that your balance exercises are consistently skipped or that your endurance is improving week by week. This insight allows you to adjust your routine as needed, ensuring you stay on track toward your fitness goals.

Using exercise tracking charts increases accountability. When you record your activities, you create a commitment to yourself. This simple act can motivate you to stick to your exercise plan, even on days when you might feel less inclined to work out. The charts also help track rest days and recovery periods, ensuring you give your body the necessary time to heal and build strength. This balance between exercise and rest is crucial for avoiding injuries and promoting long-term fitness.

To use the charts effectively, start by recording the type of exercise you performed, its duration, and the intensity. For example, if you went for a brisk walk, note the time spent walking and how intense the activity felt. This information helps you gauge your progress and make necessary adjustments. Noting any modifications or adaptations is also important. If you had to switch from walking to a seated exercise due to discomfort, record this change. Tracking these adaptations provides a comprehensive view of your fitness journey, highlighting how you adapt your routines to meet your needs.

Sample exercise tracking charts can vary depending on your preferences and fitness goals. A weekly exercise log with columns for each day allows you to record daily activities, making it easy to see your efforts at a glance. This format is particularly useful for tracking consistency and ensuring you incorporate various exercises throughout the week. A monthly overview chart offers a broader perspective, helping you track long-term progress and set larger fitness goals. This chart can be especially motivating as it shows how your efforts accumulate over time.

Customizable templates cater to specific exercise routines, allowing you to tailor the charts to your unique needs. For instance, if you focus on strength training, your chart might include sections for different muscle groups and the weights used. This level of detail helps you track improvements in strength and adjust your routine to continue challenging your muscles. Customizable templates ensure that your tracking system aligns with your fitness goals, providing a personalized approach to monitoring your progress.

The benefits of regular tracking extend beyond motivation and accountability. Consistent tracking increases adherence to exercise plans, as the visual representation of your efforts can be highly motivating. It also allows you to set and achieve specific fitness goals. For instance, you might aim to increase the duration of your walks or the number of repetitions in your strength training routine. Seeing your progress toward these goals can be incredibly rewarding and encourage you to continue pushing forward.

Enhanced understanding of personal progress and limitations is another significant benefit. By regularly reviewing your charts, you gain a clearer picture of what works for you and what doesn't. This insight helps you tailor your exercise routine to your needs, maximizing the benefits and minimizing the risk of injury. It also allows you to celebrate your achievements, no matter how small, fostering a positive mindset and reinforcing your commitment to maintaining your bone health.

Interactive Element: Sample Exercise Tracking Chart

Here is a sample weekly exercise tracking chart to help you get started. You are welcome to customize it based on your specific needs and preferences.

Weekly Exercise Log

Day	Exercise	Duration	Intensity	Notes	Rest
Monday	Walking	30 min	Medium		
Tuesday	Yoga	45 min		Chair	
Wednesday	Resistance	20 min	High	Soreness	
Thursday	Cycling	30 min	Medium		
Friday	Tai Chi	40 min	Low		
Saturday	Walking	30 min	Medium		
Sunday					X

This tracking chart includes columns for the day, exercise type, duration, intensity, any modifications or notes, and rest or recovery periods. Using this chart, you can easily monitor your weekly activities, ensuring a balanced and effective fitness routine.

By incorporating exercise tracking charts into your daily routine, you can transform your approach to fitness. These charts provide a clear visual representation of your progress, helping you stay accountable and motivated. They also offer valuable insights into your exercise patterns, allowing you to make informed adjustments and achieve your fitness goals. Whether you use a weekly log, a monthly overview, or customizable templates, tracking your exercises can lead to improved outcomes and a better understanding of your bone health journey.

10.2 MEAL PLANNING TEMPLATES

Meal planning is a fundamental aspect of maintaining bone health. By planning your meals, you ensure that your diet is balanced and rich in essential nutrients, reducing the likelihood of deficiencies that can weaken bones. Consistent nutrition is vital for seniors, as it supports bone density and overall well-being. Meal planning simplifies grocery shopping and meal preparation, making it easier to stick to a bone-healthy diet. When you have a clear plan, you can avoid last-minute unhealthy choices and ensure that your meals include the necessary vitamins and minerals for strong bones.

Different types of meal planning templates can help you organize your diet effectively. Daily meal plans are a great way to ensure that each meal and snack throughout the day contributes to your nutritional goals. These templates typically include sections for breakfast, lunch, dinner, and snacks, allowing you to plan a varied and nutrient-dense diet. Weekly meal plans are another excellent tool, offering space for grocery lists and meal preparation notes. This format helps you see the bigger picture of your dietary habits and make adjustments as needed. Monthly meal plans provide long-term dietary tracking, helping you stay consistent with your bone health goals over an extended period. These templates can include space for noting special dietary goals, such as increasing calcium intake or incorporating more leafy greens.

Using meal planning templates effectively involves incorporating various bone-healthy foods into your diet. Foods rich in calcium, such as dairy products and fortified plant-based milks, are crucial for bone formation and maintenance. Vitamin D is essential for calcium absorption, so include sources like fatty fish and fortified cereals. Magnesium, found in nuts and seeds, and vitamin K2, present in fermented foods and certain cheeses, also play vital roles in bone health. When planning your meals, aim to include a balance of these nutrients to support your bones. Preparing meals in advance can save time and make it easier to stick to your plan. For instance, you might cook a large batch of a calcium-rich casserole and portion it out for lunches throughout the week. This practice ensures that you always have a nutritious meal on hand, reducing the temptation to opt for less healthy options.

Adjusting your meal plans based on personal preferences and dietary needs is also important. If you have dietary restrictions or preferences, such as being lactose intolerant or vegetarian, tailor your meal plans to suit these needs. There are plenty of non-dairy sources of calcium, such as almonds and tofu, and plant-based sources of protein, like beans and lentils. Personalizing your meal plans ensures that you enjoy your meals and stick to your bone health goals.

Here is a sample one-week meal plan to help you get started. This plan includes recipes and a shopping list to make meal preparation straightforward.

One-Week Meal Plan

Monday

- Breakfast: Greek yogurt with mixed berries and a drizzle of honey
- Lunch: Spinach and salmon salad with lemon dressing
- Dinner: Grilled chicken with quinoa and steamed broccoli
- Snack: Almonds and dried apricots

Tuesday

- Breakfast: Oatmeal with sliced bananas and walnuts
- Lunch: Lentil soup with a side of whole-grain bread
- Dinner: Baked tofu with brown rice and sautéed kale
- Snack: Cottage cheese with pineapple

Wednesday

- Breakfast: Smoothie with fortified plant milk, spinach, and frozen berries
- Lunch: Chickpea and avocado wrap
- Dinner: Baked salmon with sweet potato and green beans
- Snack: Carrot sticks with hummus

Thursday

- Breakfast: Scrambled eggs with spinach and whole-grain toast
- Lunch: Quinoa salad with roasted vegetables
- Dinner: Turkey chili with a side of cornbread
- Snack: Greek yogurt with a handful of mixed nuts

Friday

- Breakfast: Smoothie bowl with fortified plant milk, banana, and granola
- Lunch: Tuna salad with mixed greens and balsamic vinaigrette
- Dinner: Stir-fried tofu with brown rice and mixed vegetables
- Snack: Apple slices with almond butter

Saturday

- Breakfast: Whole-grain pancakes with fresh fruit
- Lunch: Black bean and corn salad with lime dressing
- Dinner: Grilled shrimp with quinoa and asparagus
- Snack: Cheese and whole-grain crackers

Sunday

- Breakfast: Fortified plant milk smoothie with protein powder, spinach, and berries
- Lunch: Tomato and basil soup with a side of whole-grain bread
- Dinner: Chicken and vegetable stir-fry with brown rice
- Snack: Fresh fruit salad

To assist you in creating your own meal plans, here is a blank template.

Blank Meal Planning Template

Monday

- Breakfast:
- Lunch:
- Dinner:
- Snack:

Tuesday

- Breakfast:
- Lunch:
- Dinner:
- Snack:

Wednesday

- Breakfast:
- Lunch:
- Dinner:
- Snack:

Thursday

- Breakfast:
- Lunch:
- Dinner:
- Snack:

Friday

- Breakfast:
- Lunch:
- Dinner:
- Snack:

Saturday

- Breakfast:
- Lunch:
- Dinner:
- Snack:

Sunday

- Breakfast:
- Lunch:
- Dinner:
- Snack:

For those who prefer long-term planning, a monthly calendar can help track special dietary goals and ensure consistency. This calendar can include space for noting goals like "Increase calcium intake" or "Incorporate more leafy greens."

Monthly Meal Planning Calendar

Week - Goal \ Notes

Week 1 - Increase calcium intake \ Add more dairy and leafy greens

Week 2 - Reduce sugar intake \ Avoid processed foods and sweets

Week 3 - Incorporate more vegetables \ Add a vegetable to every meal

Week 4 - Try new recipes \ Experiment with new healthy recipes

Using these templates, you can plan your meals effectively, ensuring a balanced and nutrient-rich diet that supports your bone health.

10.3 SUPPLEMENT DOSAGE SCHEDULES

Maintaining a consistent supplement schedule is crucial for bone health. It ensures you receive an adequate intake of essential nutrients like calcium, vitamin D, and magnesium. These nutrients play critical roles in maintaining bone density and strength. Missing doses or taking supplements erratically can lead to deficiencies, weakening your bones over time. A well-structured supplement schedule helps prevent missed doses and avoids over-supplementation, which can have adverse effects. For instance, excessive calcium intake can lead to kidney stones, while too much vitamin D can cause toxicity. Consistency in taking supplements supports overall health and well-being, providing a steady supply of the nutrients your bones need to stay strong.

There are various types of supplement dosage schedules you can use to stay on track. Daily schedules are straightforward and involve taking specific supplements at designated times each day.

This method is particularly effective for supplements that need to be taken multiple times a day, such as calcium, which is best absorbed in smaller doses. Weekly charts offer a broader overview, allowing you to track your supplement intake throughout the week. These charts can include space for notes on how you feel or any side effects you experience. Monthly logs provide a long-term perspective, helping you maintain consistency over weeks and months. This approach is especially useful for tracking supplements that you may not need to take daily, but still require regular monitoring.

Creating a personalized supplement schedule involves several steps. First, determine the best time of day to take each supplement. Some, like calcium, are best taken with meals to enhance absorption and minimize gastrointestinal discomfort. Others, like magnesium, can be taken before bed as they promote relaxation and improve sleep quality. Next, consider any interactions with medications or other supplements you are taking. For example, calcium can interfere with the absorption of certain medications, so it's important to space them out. Adjusting doses based on individual needs and health conditions is also crucial. Your healthcare provider can offer guidance on the appropriate dosages for your specific situation, ensuring you get the maximum benefit without overdoing it.

Here's a sample daily supplement schedule to help you get started. In the morning, you might take a multivitamin with breakfast, ensuring you get a broad range of nutrients to start your day. Mid-morning, you could take a calcium supplement with a snack to aid absorption. At lunchtime, a vitamin D supplement can be beneficial, especially if you have limited sun exposure. In the afternoon, consider taking magnesium, which can help with muscle function and relaxation. Finally, an evening dose of calcium before bed can provide your bones with a steady supply of this critical mineral overnight. This schedule ensures you spread out your nutrient intake, enhancing absorption and minimizing the risk of side effects.

For those who prefer a weekly chart, consider using a format that allows you to track your supplement intake each day. This chart can include columns for each day of the week, with rows for different supplements. You can note the time you took each supplement and any additional comments or side effects. This format provides a comprehensive overview of your supplement regimen, making it easier to identify patterns and adjust as needed. For instance, if you notice that taking magnesium in the morning makes you feel drowsy, you can adjust your schedule to take it in the evening instead. This flexibility ensures you get the most benefit from your supplements while minimizing any negative effects.

A monthly log offers a long-term perspective, helping you maintain consistency over weeks and months. This log can include space for tracking your supplement intake, as well as notes on any changes in your health or how you feel. For example, you might note improvements in your energy levels or reductions in joint pain, providing valuable feedback on the effectiveness of your supplement regimen. This long-term tracking helps you stay committed to your bone health goals, providing a clear record of your efforts and progress.

Interactive Element: Sample Supplement Dosage Schedule

Here is a customizable template to help you create your own supplement schedule.

Time	Supplement	Dosage	Notes
Morning	Multivitamin	1 tablet	Breakfast
Mid-Morning	Calcium	500 mg	With snack
Lunch	Vit D	1000 IU	Lunch meal
Afternoon	Magnesium	250 mg	With snack
Evening	Calcium	500 mg	Before bed

Using this template, you can design a supplement schedule that fits seamlessly into your daily routine. This consistency ensures you receive the nutrients your bones need to stay strong and healthy. Regular tracking and adjustments based on your needs and health conditions make this approach both effective and sustainable.

10.4 WEEKLY PROGRESS JOURNALS

Tracking your progress in a weekly journal can profoundly impact how you manage your bone health. It serves as a personal record of your achievements and challenges, providing a tangible way to see your efforts and improvements over time. This record encourages self-reflection and goal setting, allowing you to identify what works for you and where you need to make changes. It becomes easier to spot trends and areas for improvement, whether it's realizing you need more rest days or noticing that a particular exercise routine is yielding great results.

Weekly progress journals come in various formats, each designed to meet different needs. A simple weekly log with space for daily entries can help you keep track of your daily activities and how they affect your bone health. This straightforward approach allows you to jot down quick notes about your exercise, diet, and any symptoms you might experience. For those who prefer a more reflective approach, detailed journals with prompts for reflection and goal setting are ideal. These journals guide you through the process of thinking about your week, what you accomplished, and what you can improve. Interactive journals that track multiple aspects of health, such as exercise, nutrition, and mental well-being, offer a comprehensive view of your overall progress.

To use a progress journal effectively, set aside a specific time each week for journaling. This dedicated time ensures you consistently reflect on your week and make thoughtful entries. Be honest and detailed in your entries; this authenticity will make your journal a valuable tool for tracking your progress and making necessary adjustments. Use your journal to celebrate successes, no matter how small. Recognizing these achievements can boost your motivation and encourage you to keep going. Additionally, plan for future goals based on your reflections. If you notice that you consistently struggle with a particular exercise, set a goal to improve in that area.

Here's a simple weekly log to help you get started. This log includes columns for each day, where you can note your activities, how you felt, and any changes or observations. For example, Monday might include a note about a morning walk, how your joints felt afterward, and any modifications you made to your routine. This simple format helps you quickly capture the key elements of your day, making it easy to review and adjust as needed.

For those who prefer a more detailed approach, consider a journal with prompts for reflecting on your progress and setting new goals. These prompts might ask you to think about what went well this week, what challenges you faced, and how you can address them moving forward. This reflective practice helps you gain more in-depth insights into your bone health management and make more informed decisions about your routine.

An interactive journal provides space for tracking multiple aspects of health, such as exercise, nutrition, and overall well-being. This comprehensive approach ensures you capture a complete picture of your health, making it easier to see how different factors interact and affect your bone health. For instance, you might notice that on days when you eat particularly well, you also feel more energetic and perform better in your exercises. This insight can help you make more informed choices about your diet and exercise routine.

To assist you in creating your own progress journal, here's a customizable template.

Simple Weekly Log

Day	Activity	Observations
Monday	Morning walk	Joint pain reduced
Tuesday	Yoga	Relaxed – Used chair
Wednesday	Resistance training	Mild muscle soreness
Thursday	Cycling	Energetic
Friday	Tai Chi	Balanced and calm
Saturday	Gardening	Slight back pain
Sunday	Rest day	Refreshed

Detailed Journal with Prompts

- What went well this week?
- What challenges did I face?

- How did I address these challenges?
- What can I improve next week?
- What new goals do I want to set?

By using this template, you can create a progress journal that fits your needs and preferences. This practice will help you stay on track with your bone health goals, providing a clear record of your achievements and challenges. Regular journaling encourages self-reflection and goal setting, helping you identify trends and areas for improvement. Whether you prefer a simple log, a detailed journal, or an interactive format, progress journaling can enhance your bone health management and support your overall well-being.

Chapter 10 has covered tools and strategies to help you monitor and manage your bone health effectively. These tools provide a structured approach to tracking your progress, ensuring you stay committed to your goals. As we move forward, we will explore more practical tips and strategies to support your journey toward better bone health.

Spread the Word: Healthy Bones Are Linked to Good Overall Health

I hope this book has ticked all the boxes when it comes to strengthening your bones and staying motivated to pursue a healthy lifestyle. You have seen how all the strategies I have suggested—including nutrition, exercise, stress management, and the use of interactive tools—are part of a holistic plan of action for good bone and general health. All these approaches, taken together, will not only keep the onslaught of osteoporosis at bay but also help you feel stronger, more energetic, and—dare I say—happier!

A wealth of studies have shown that simply getting a good night's sleep and eating gut-healthy foods can significantly impact your mental health. And of course, staying mentally sharp is key if you wish to maintain your motivation and commitment to caring for your bones.

You have so much to do—from shopping for healthy foods to harnessing the latest tools to track your progress. However, before you go, please share your opinion of this book with people who are keen to find a simple-to-follow, holistic approach to good bone health.

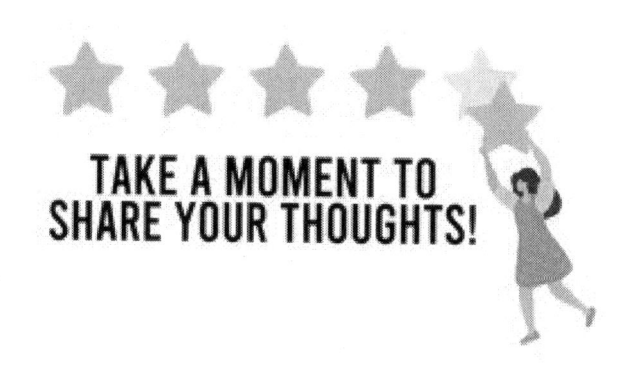

TAKE A MOMENT TO SHARE YOUR THOUGHTS!

Let others know the choices they make now will have a tremendous impact on their health and enjoyment of life in their later years!

Scan the QR code below

CONCLUSION

As we come to the end of this journey, it is vital to emphasize the profound importance of bone health. Our bones are the foundation of our physical existence, providing structure, protection, and the ability to move freely. As we age, maintaining strong and healthy bones becomes paramount to preserving our quality of life and independence.

Throughout this book, we have delved into various aspects of bone health, offering a comprehensive guide tailored specifically for seniors. We began by understanding the anatomy and functions of bones, highlighting the differences between osteoporosis and osteopenia, and exploring the impact of arthritis on bone health. We then discussed the science behind bone density and the critical role it plays in overall bone strength.

Our exploration continued with medical options and explanations, guiding you through bone density scans, prescription medications, and non-pharmaceutical interventions. We provided detailed nutritional guidance, emphasizing the importance of calcium, vitamin D, protein, and other essential nutrients. We also examined the role of supplements and offered practical tips for incorporating them into your daily routine.

Exercise is a cornerstone of bone health, and we dedicated an entire chapter to detailed exercise routines, ranging from beginner to elite levels. We shared personal stories and testimonials to inspire and motivate you, showing that it is possible to overcome bone health challenges with determination and the right strategies.

We addressed common pain points and questions, offering solutions for safe exercises, navigating nutritional needs, managing limited mobility, and effective supplementation. Lastly, we equipped you with interactive tools and elements to track your progress and stay consistent in your bone health journey.

The key takeaways from this book are clear: maintaining strong bones requires a multifaceted approach that includes proper nutrition, regular exercise, medical interventions when necessary, and a commitment to holistic health practices. By integrating these strategies into your daily life, you can significantly improve your bone health and overall well-being.

Now, it is time for action. I encourage you to implement the strategies discussed in this book. Start with small, manageable changes and gradually build upon them. Incorporate weight-bearing exercises into your routine, ensure you are getting enough calcium and vitamin D, and take the necessary supplements to fill any nutritional gaps. Stay consistent with your efforts, track your progress, and celebrate your achievements along the way.

Remember, taking care of your bones is not just about preventing fractures or managing pain. It is about empowering yourself to lead an active, independent, and fulfilling life. Your bone health journey is a lifelong commitment, but the rewards are immeasurable.

As a retired sports chiropractor with over 40 years of experience, I have witnessed firsthand the transformative power of these strategies. I have seen patients like Jack, George, Helen, Doris, Harold, Martha, Irene, Jane, Mark, Linda, Rachel, and John reclaim their lives and thrive despite their bone health challenges. Their stories are a testament to the resilience of the human spirit and the effectiveness of a comprehensive bone health approach.

In closing, I want to leave you with this thought: your bones are your lifelong companions. Treat them with the care and respect they deserve. By doing so, you will enhance your physical health and enrich your overall quality of life. Embrace the journey, stay committed, and take proactive steps to ensure your bones remain strong and healthy for years to come.

Thank you for allowing me to be a part of your bone health journey. I hope this book has provided you with valuable insights, practical tips, and the motivation to take charge of your bone health. Wishing you strength, vitality, and a life filled with joy and independence.

Dr. K.D. Christensen

REFERENCES

Biology of Bone Tissue: Structure, Function, and Factors That ... https://www.ncbi.nlm.nih.gov/pmc/articles/PMC4515490/#:

What is the difference between osteopenia and osteoporosis? https://www.medicalnewstoday.com/articles/osteopenia-vs-osteoporosis#:

What Are Common Types of Arthritis in Seniors? https://www.visitingangels.com/knowledge-center/senior-health-and-well-being/common-types-of-arthritis-in-seniors/19401

Aging and bone loss: new insights for the clinician - PMC https://www.ncbi.nlm.nih.gov/pmc/articles/PMC3383520/

Bone Density Scan (DEXA or DXA) https://www.radiologyinfo.org/en/info/dexa

Osteoporosis treatment: Medications can help https://www.mayoclinic.org/diseases-conditions/osteoporosis/in-depth/osteoporosis-treatment/art-20046869

Bone Mineral Density Tests: What the Numbers Mean https://www.niams.nih.gov/health-topics/bone-mineral-density-tests-what-numbers-mean

Non-pharmacological management of osteoporosis https://www.ncbi.nlm.nih.gov/pmc/articles/PMC3186889/

Top 15 Calcium-Rich Foods (Many Are Nondairy) https://www.healthline.com/nutrition/15-calcium-rich-foods

How Much Calcium Do Adults Over 55 Need? https://newsnetwork.mayoclinic.org/discussion/calcium-intake-for-adults-over-age-55/

Calcium and Vitamin D: Important for Bone Health | NIAMS https://www.niams.nih.gov/health-topics/calcium-and-vitamin-d-important-bone-health#:

Protein Consumption and the Elderly: What Is the Optimal ... https://www.ncbi.nlm.nih.gov/pmc/articles/PMC4924200/

Dietary Supplements for Older Adults https://www.nia.nih.gov/health/vitamins-and-supplements/dietary-supplements-older-adults

Choosing a calcium supplement - Harvard Health https://www.health.harvard.edu/nutrition/choosing-a-calcium-supplement#:

Effectiveness of vitamin D2 compared with vitamin D3 ... https://www.ncbi.nlm.nih.gov/pmc/articles/PMC9372493/

What to Know About Multivitamins for Seniors https://www.webmd.com/healthy-aging/what-to-know-about-multivitamins-for-seniors

Exercise for Your Bone Health | NIAMS https://www.niams.nih.gov/health-topics/exercise-your-bone-health

REFERENCES

Slowing bone loss with weight-bearing exercise https://www.health.harvard.edu/staying-healthy/slowing-bone-loss-with-weight-bearing-exercise

Eight chair exercises for older adults with limited mobility https://www.caregiversolutions.ca/health-and-wellness/eight-chair-exercises-for-older-adults-with-limited-mobility/

Growing Stronger - Strength Training for Older Adults https://www.cdc.gov/physicalactivity/downloads/growing_stronger.pdf

Exercise for Healthy Aging - SMART Goal & FITT Principle https://www.healthedpartners.org/ceu/pa-healthyaging/Create_Healthy_Aging_Exercise_Program.pdf

Bone health: Tips to keep your bones healthy https://www.mayoclinic.org/healthy-lifestyle/adult-health/in-depth/bone-health/art-20045060

Artificial Intelligence Tools for Managing Osteoporosis - PMC https://www.ncbi.nlm.nih.gov/pmc/articles/PMC9999362/

Fall prevention: Simple tips to prevent falls https://www.mayoclinic.org/healthy-lifestyle/healthy-aging/in-depth/fall-prevention/art-20047358

Interaction of Nutrition and Exercise on Bone and Muscle https://www.ncbi.nlm.nih.gov/pmc/articles/PMC6587895/

Impacts of Psychological Stress on Osteoporosis https://www.ncbi.nlm.nih.gov/pmc/articles/PMC6465575/

The Importance of the Circadian System & Sleep for Bone ... https://www.ncbi.nlm.nih.gov/pmc/articles/PMC5994176/

Alcohol and Other Factors Affecting Osteoporosis Risk in ... https://www.ncbi.nlm.nih.gov/pmc/articles/PMC6676684/

Patient Story - Jane Pittadaki https://www.osteoporosis.foundation/patients/patient-stories/story-jane-pittadaki

Journey with osteoporosis. - Bone Health and O... https://healthunlocked.com/bonehealth/posts/141050627/journey-with-osteoporosis.

30-Day Exercise Challenge for Arthritis https://www.arthritisresearch.ca/30-day-exercise-challenge-for-arthritis/

OSTEOPOROSIS SERIES: RACHEL WILLIAMS (Nutrition ... https://www.youtube.com/watch?v=n9irv4p1Qh4

6 Best Balance Exercises for Seniors to Improve Stability https://www.silversneakers.com/blog/balance-exercises-seniors/

Optimizing bone health in older adults: the importance ... https://www.ncbi.nlm.nih.gov/pmc/articles/PMC2907525/

10 Adaptive Disability Fitness Equipment Recommendations https://www.theptdc.com/articles/disability-fitness

Osteoporosis and supplements for bone health https://newsnetwork.mayoclinic.org/discussion/mayo-clinic-q-and-a-osteoporosis-and-supplements-for-bone-health/

The Best Fitness Trackers for Seniors https://regencyoaksseniorliving.com/blog/fitness-trackers-for-seniors/

Your 7-Day Osteoporosis Diet Plan https://www.healthline.com/health/managing-osteoporosis/7-day-osteoporosis-diet-plan

Calcium and calcium supplements: Achieving the right ... https://www.mayoclinic.org/healthy-lifestyle/nutrition-and-healthy-eating/in-depth/calcium-supplements/art-20047097

Writing Your Wellness Story: Creating a Personal Progress ... https://seniorfitnessfinder.com/fitness-finder-on-fitness/writing-your-wellness-story-creating-a-personal-progress-journal-for-senior-fitness

Made in the USA
Columbia, SC
05 February 2025